Historic Flash

Spider Webb

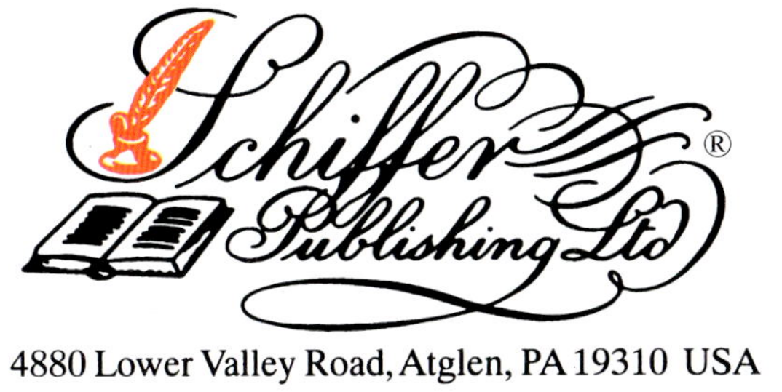

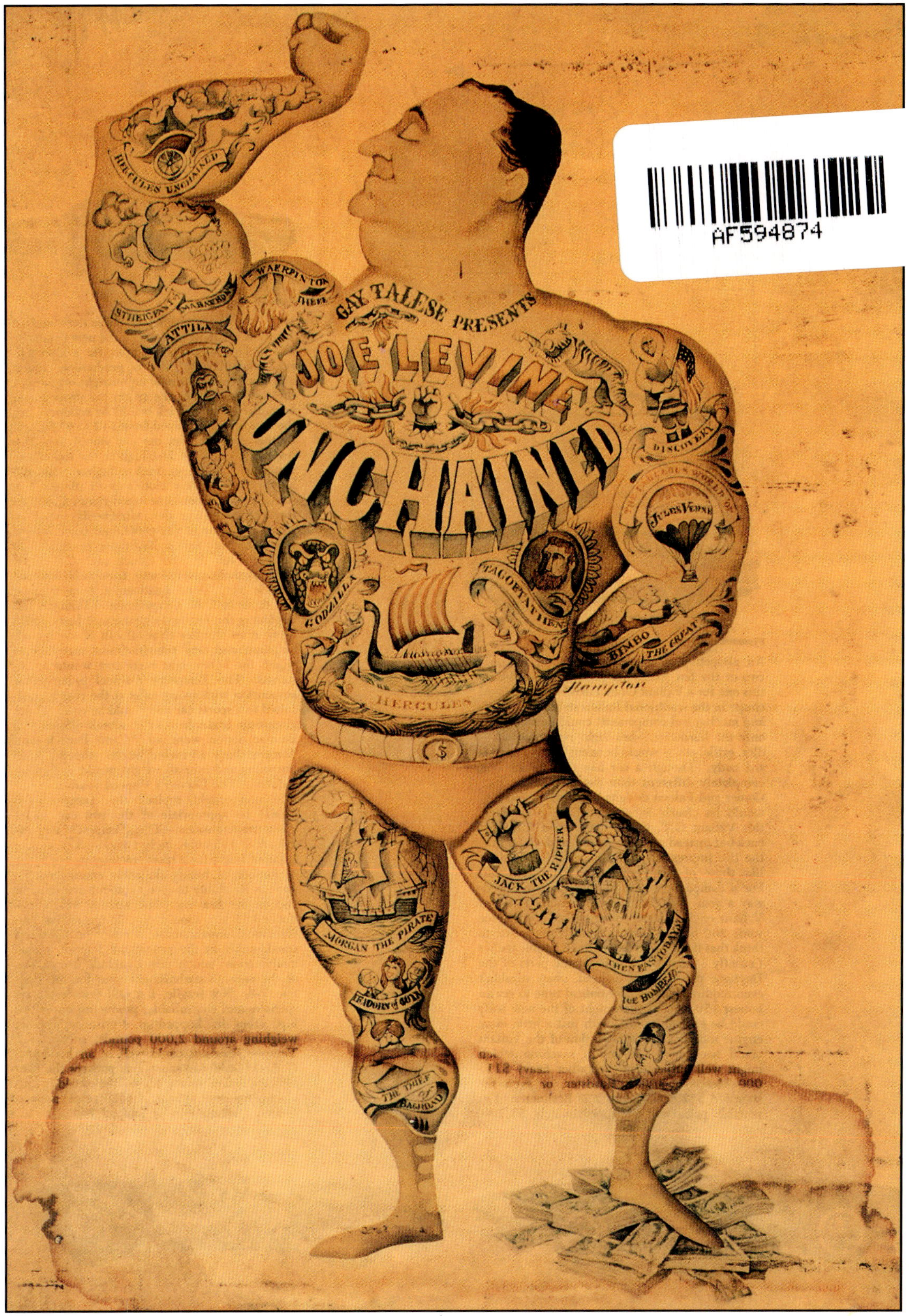

4880 Lower Valley Road, Atglen, PA 19310 USA

Library of Congress Control Number: 2001099724

Designed by Bonnie M. Hensley
Cover design by Bruce Waters
Type set in Futura HvBT/Zurich BT

ISBN: 978-0-7643-1606-7
Printed in China

Schiffer Books are available at special discounts for bulk purchases for sales promotions or premiums. Special editions, including personalized covers, corporate imprints, and excerpts can be created in large quantities for special needs. For more information contact the publisher:

Published by Schiffer Publishing Ltd.
4880 Lower Valley Road
Atglen, PA 19310
Phone: (610) 593-1777; Fax: (610) 593-2002
E-mail: Info@schifferbooks.com

For the largest selection of fine reference books on this and related subjects, please visit our website at **www.schifferbooks.com**
We are always looking for people to write books on new and related subjects. If you have an idea for a book, please contact us at proposals@schifferbooks.com

This book may be purchased from the publisher.
Include $5.00 for shipping.
Please try your bookstore first.
You may write for a free catalog.

In Europe, Schiffer books are distributed by
Bushwood Books
6 Marksbury Ave.
Kew Gardens
Surrey TW9 4JF England
Phone: 44 (0) 20 8392 8585; Fax: 44 (0) 20 8392 9876
E-mail: info@bushwoodbooks.co.uk
Website: www.bushwoodbooks.co.uk

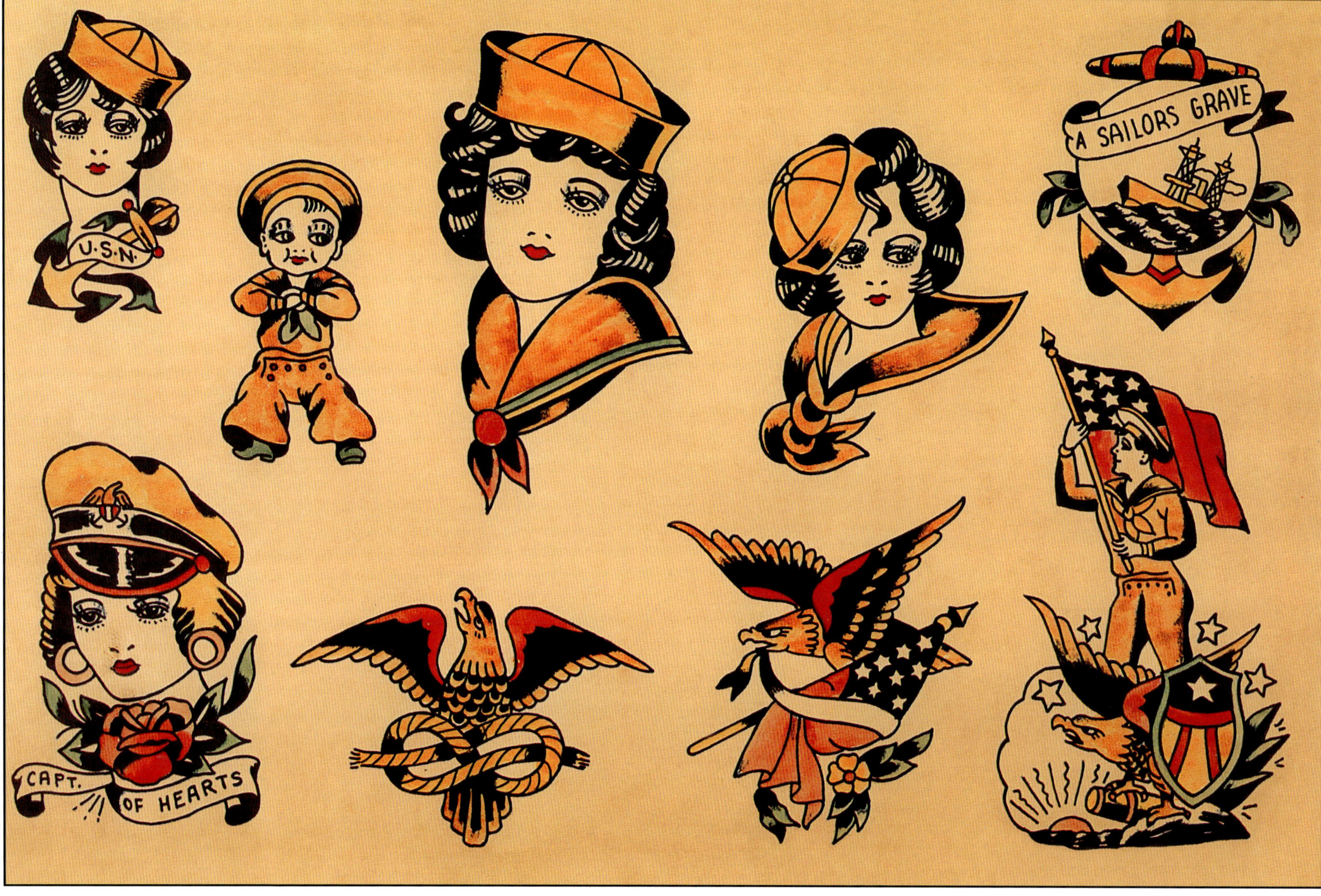

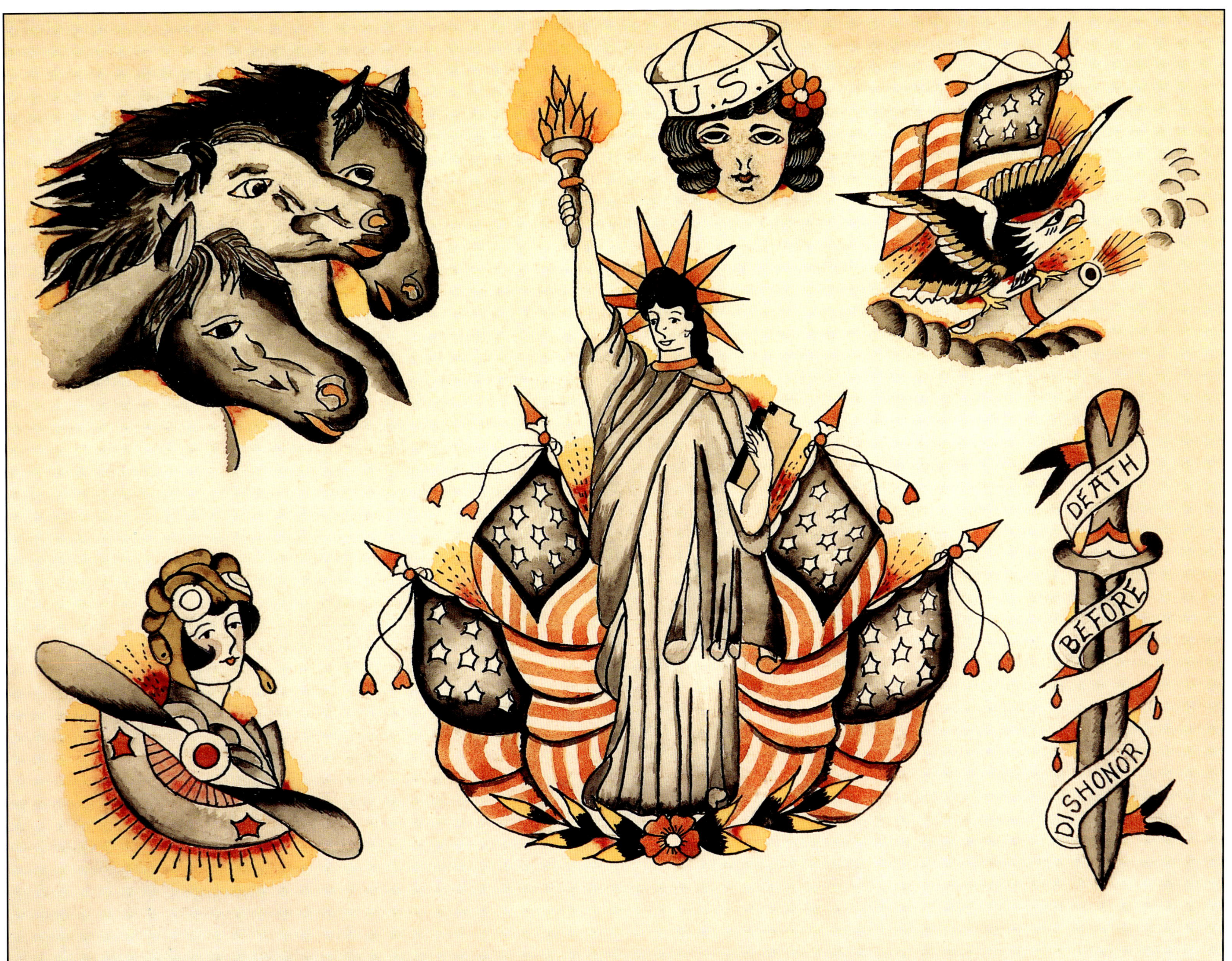
U.S.N.
DEATH
BEFORE
DISHONOR

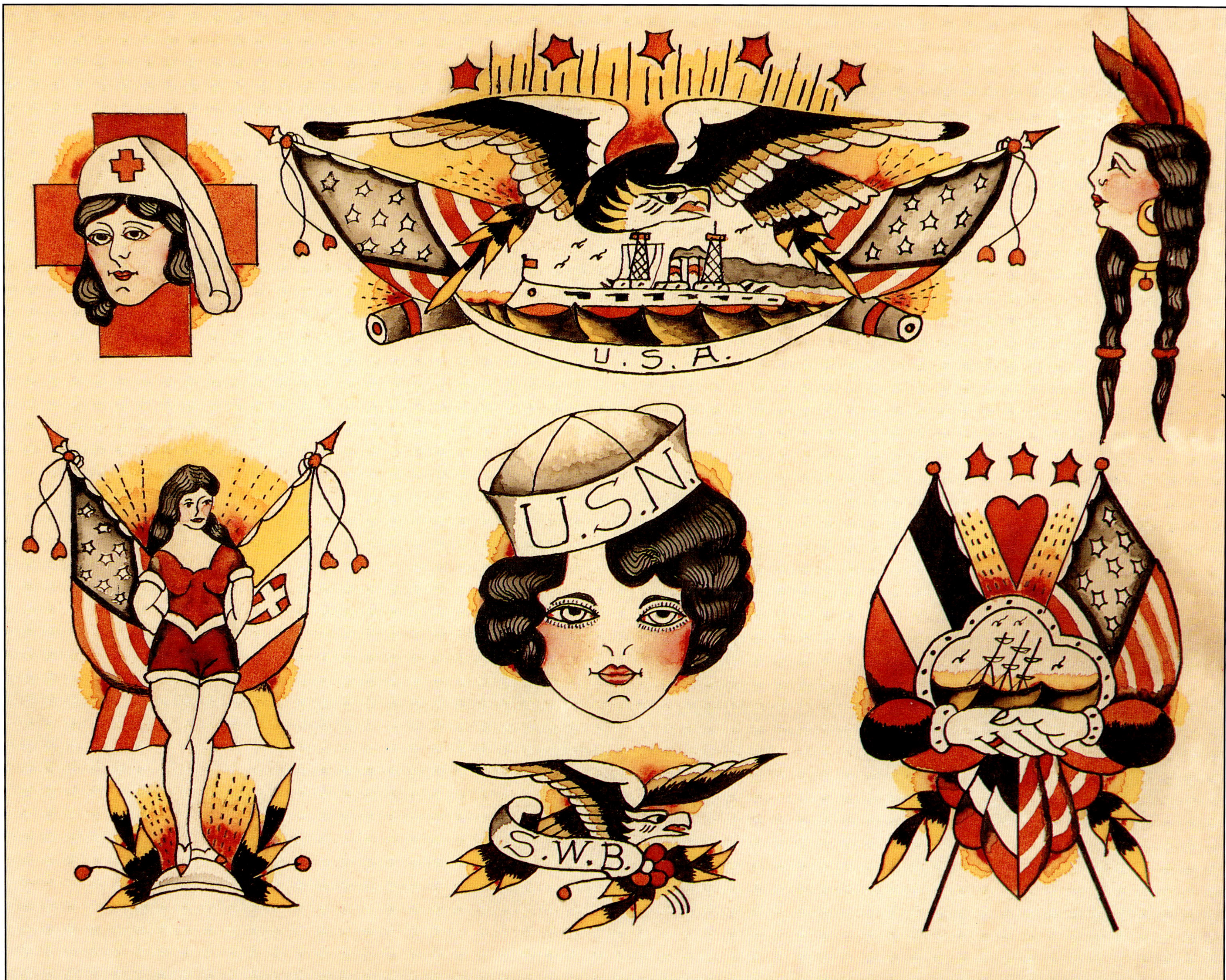
U.S.A.
U.S.N.
S.W.B.

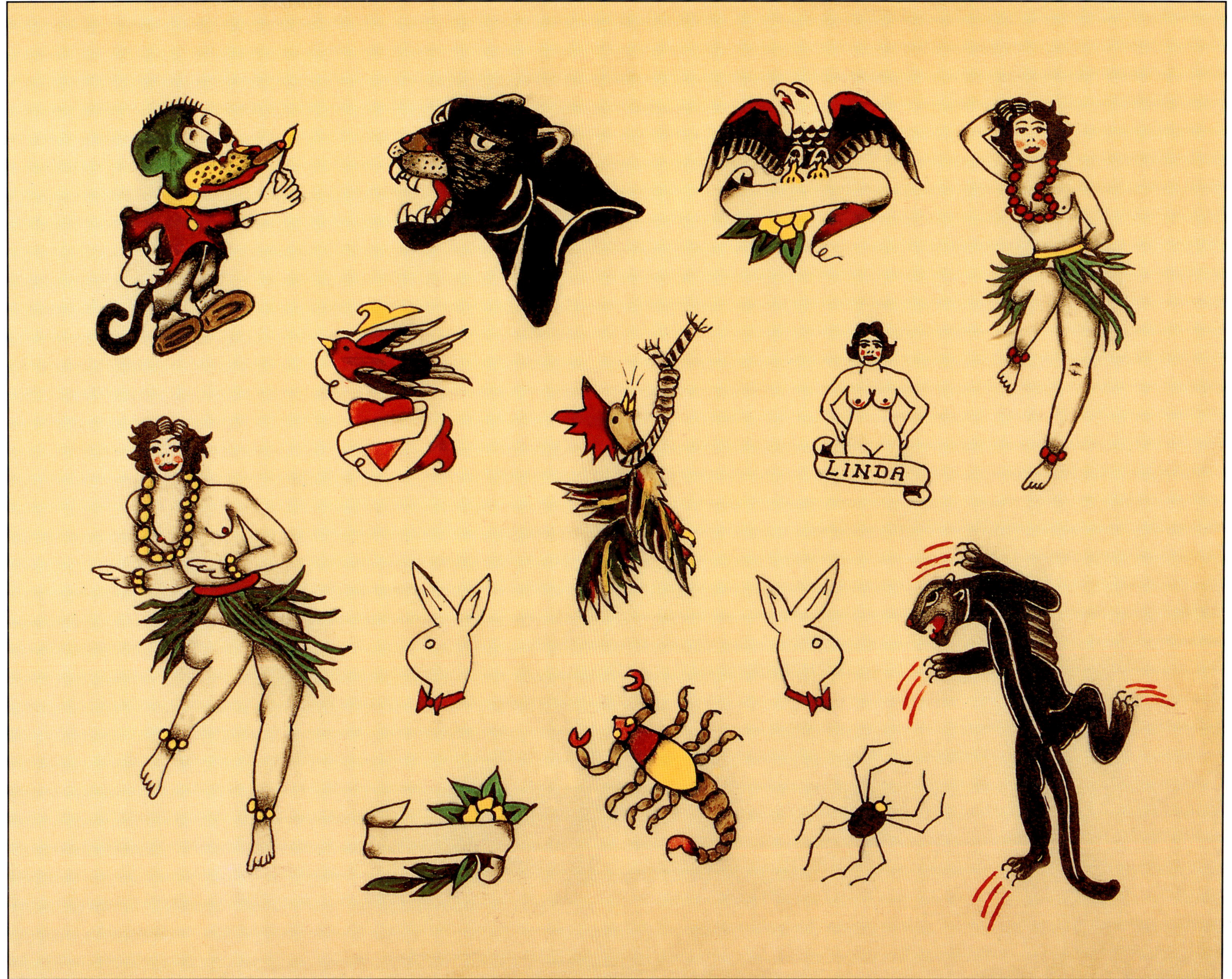
LINDA

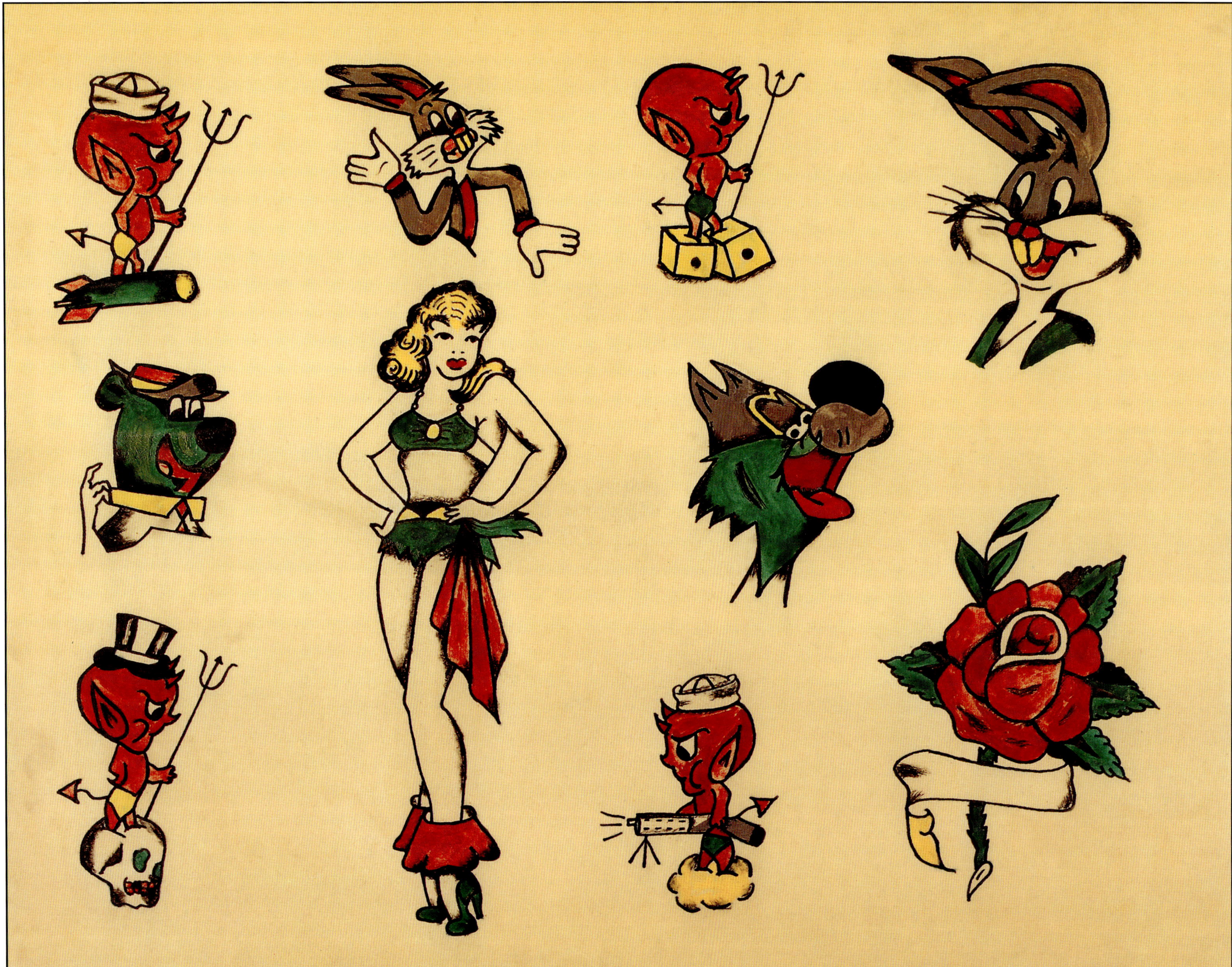

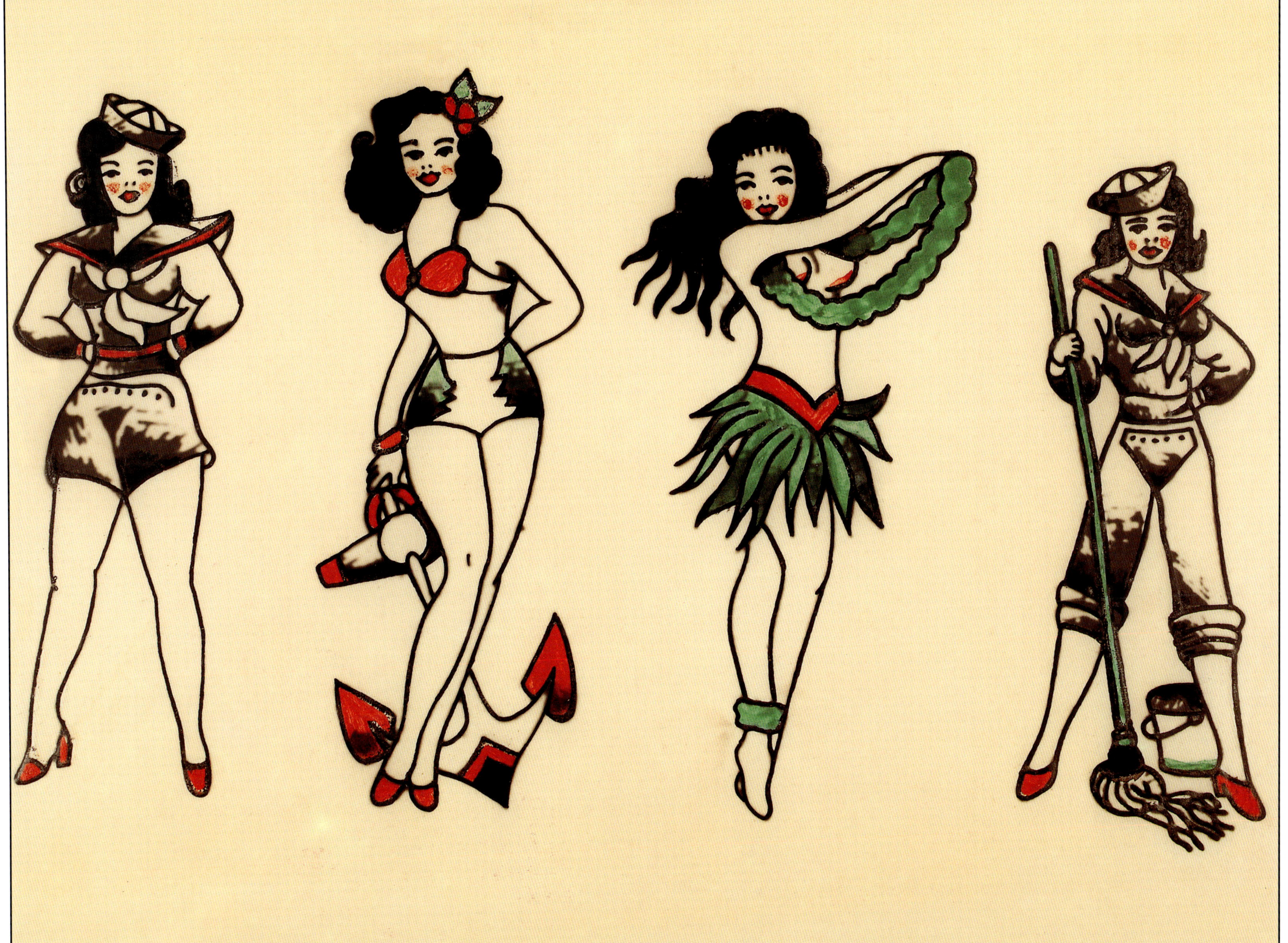

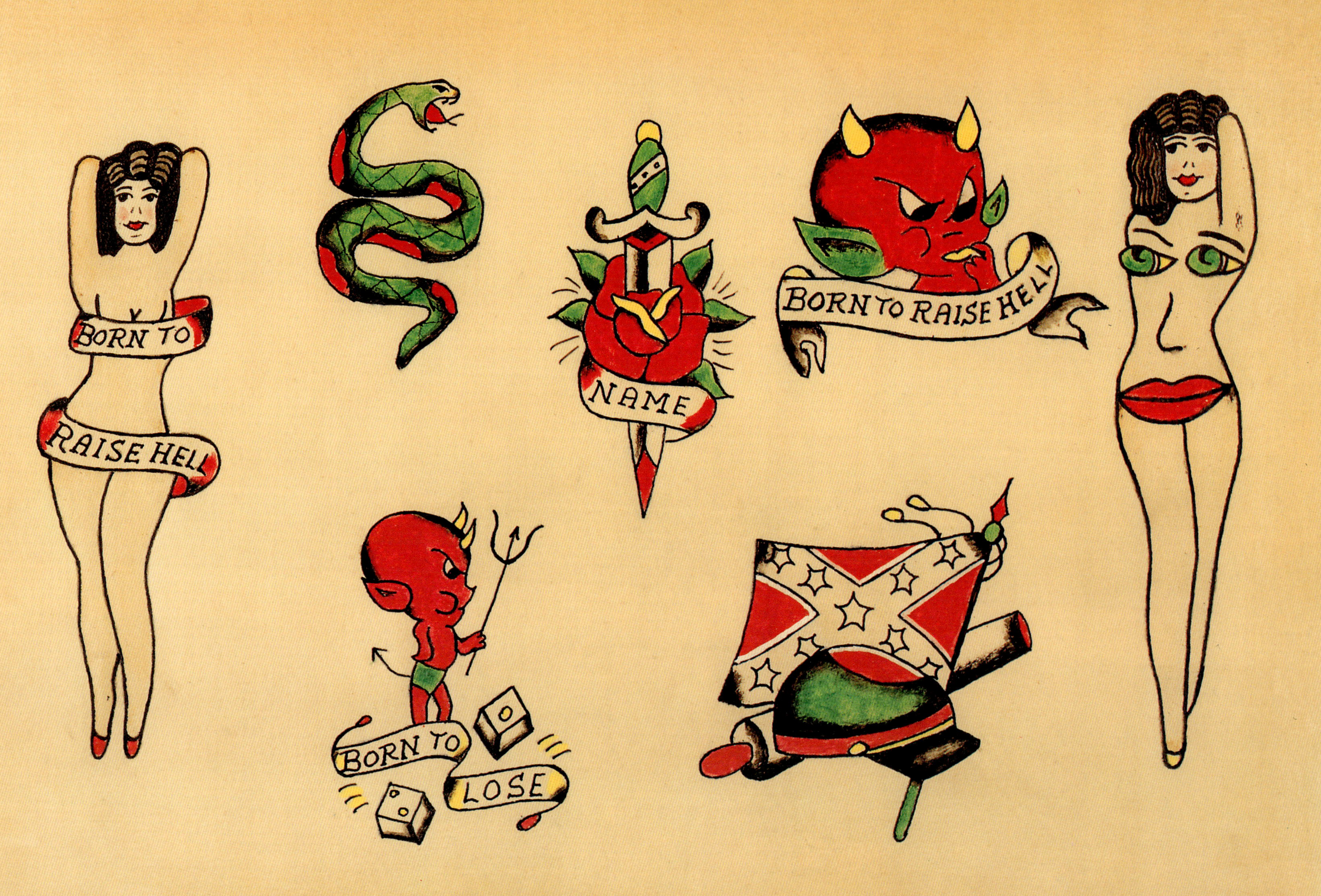
BORN TO
RAISE HELL
NAME
BORN TO RAISE HELL
BORN TO
LOSE

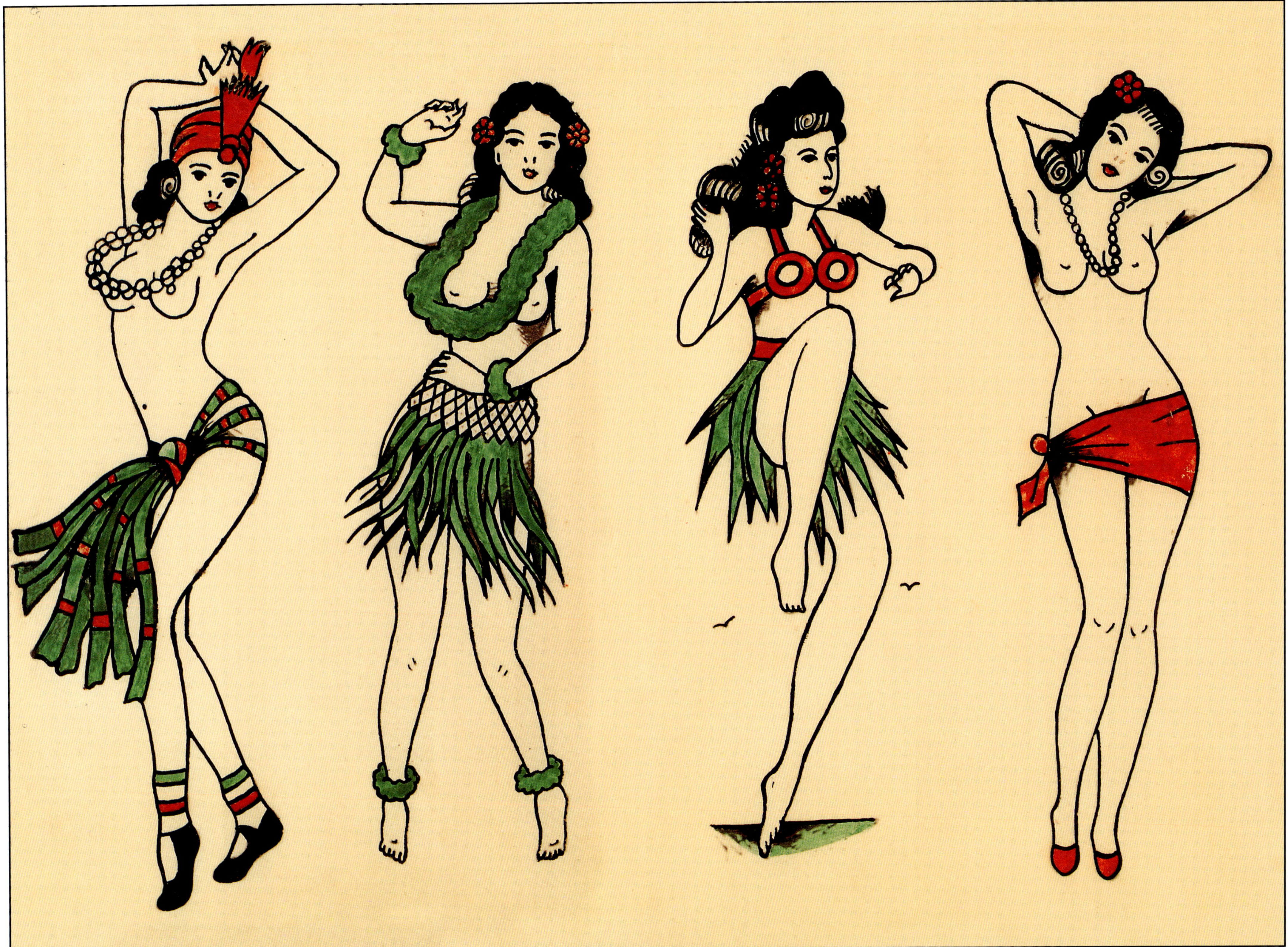

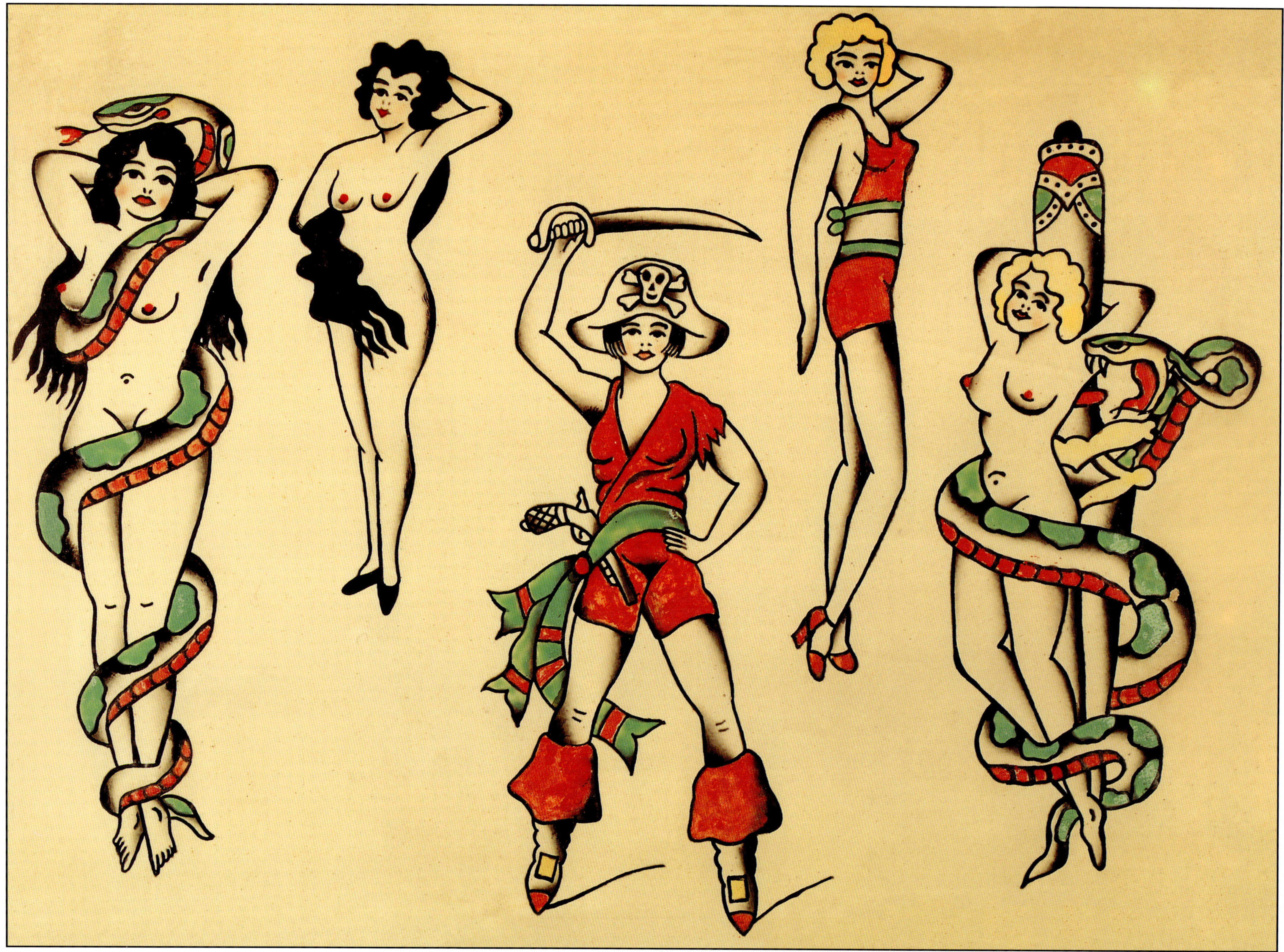

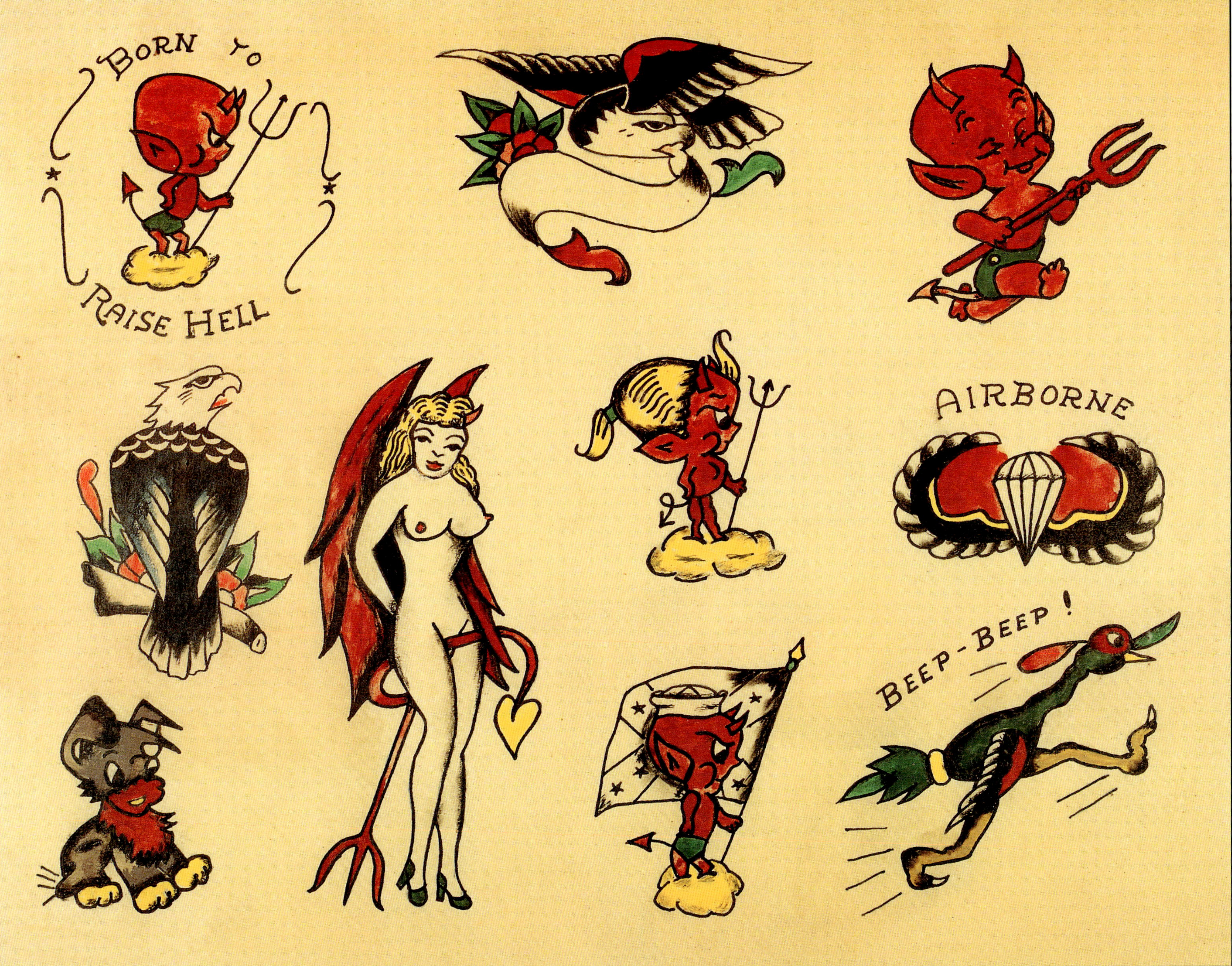
BORN TO
RAISE HELL
AIRBORNE
BEEP-BEEP!

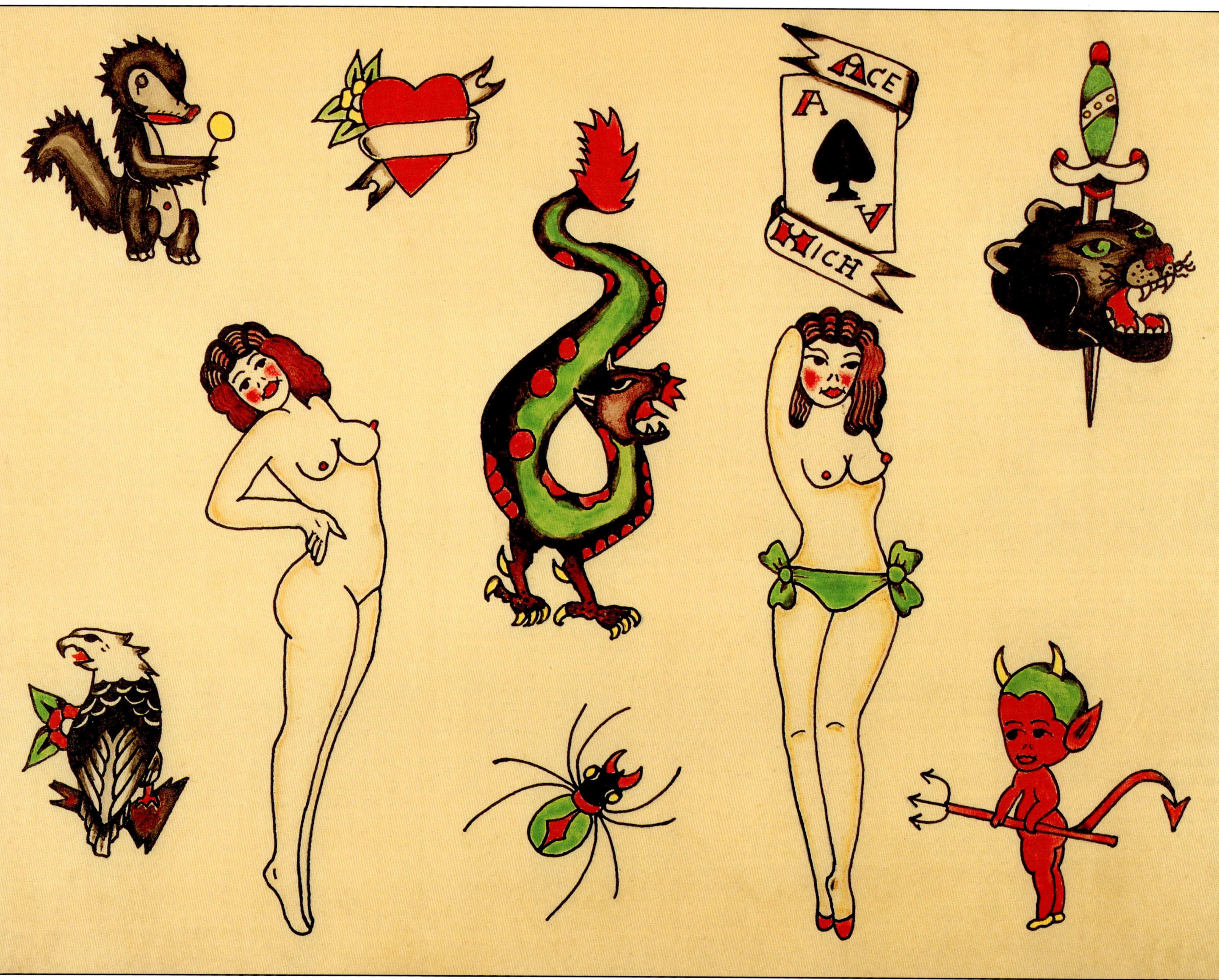
ACE
A
A
HICH

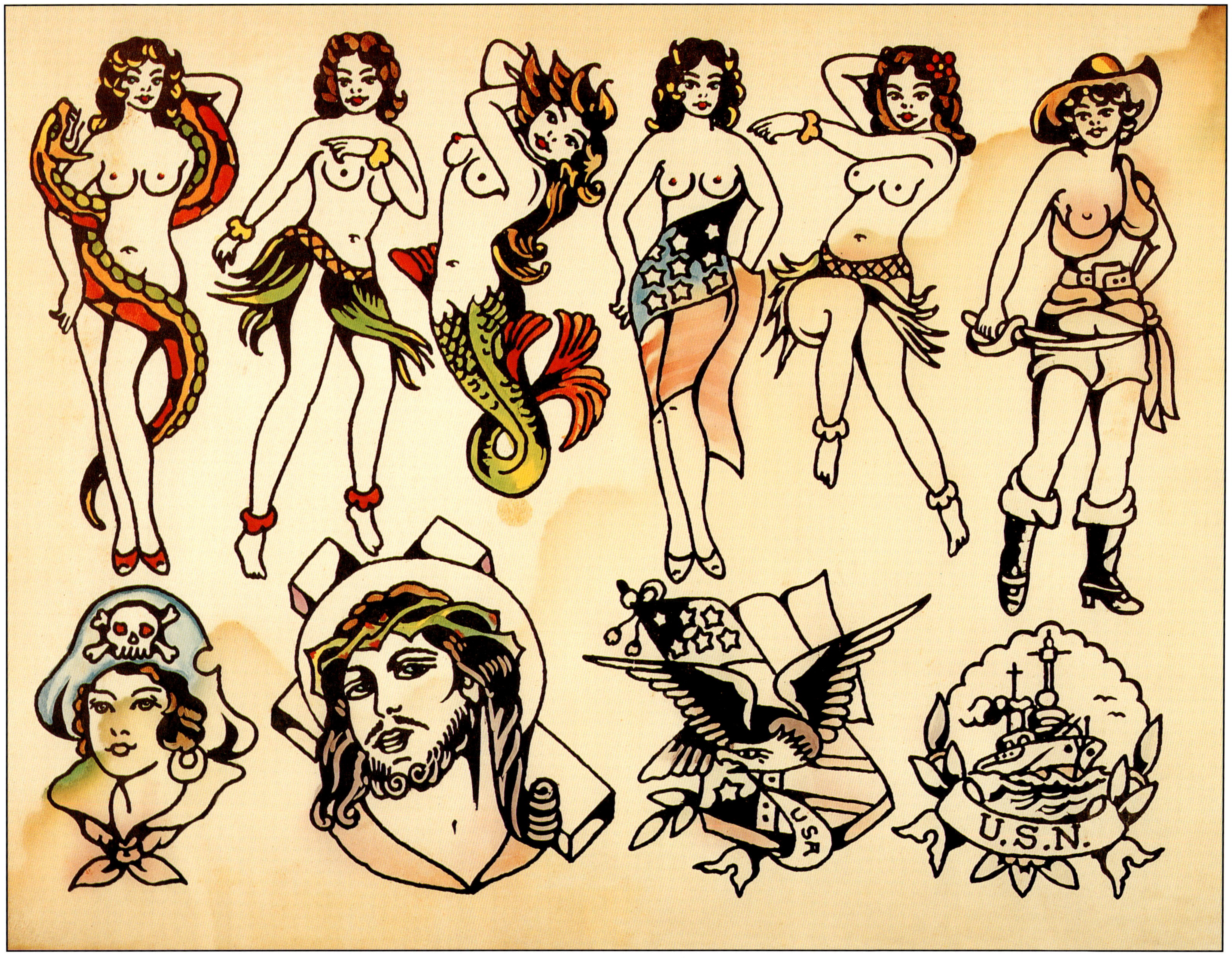
USA
U.S.N.

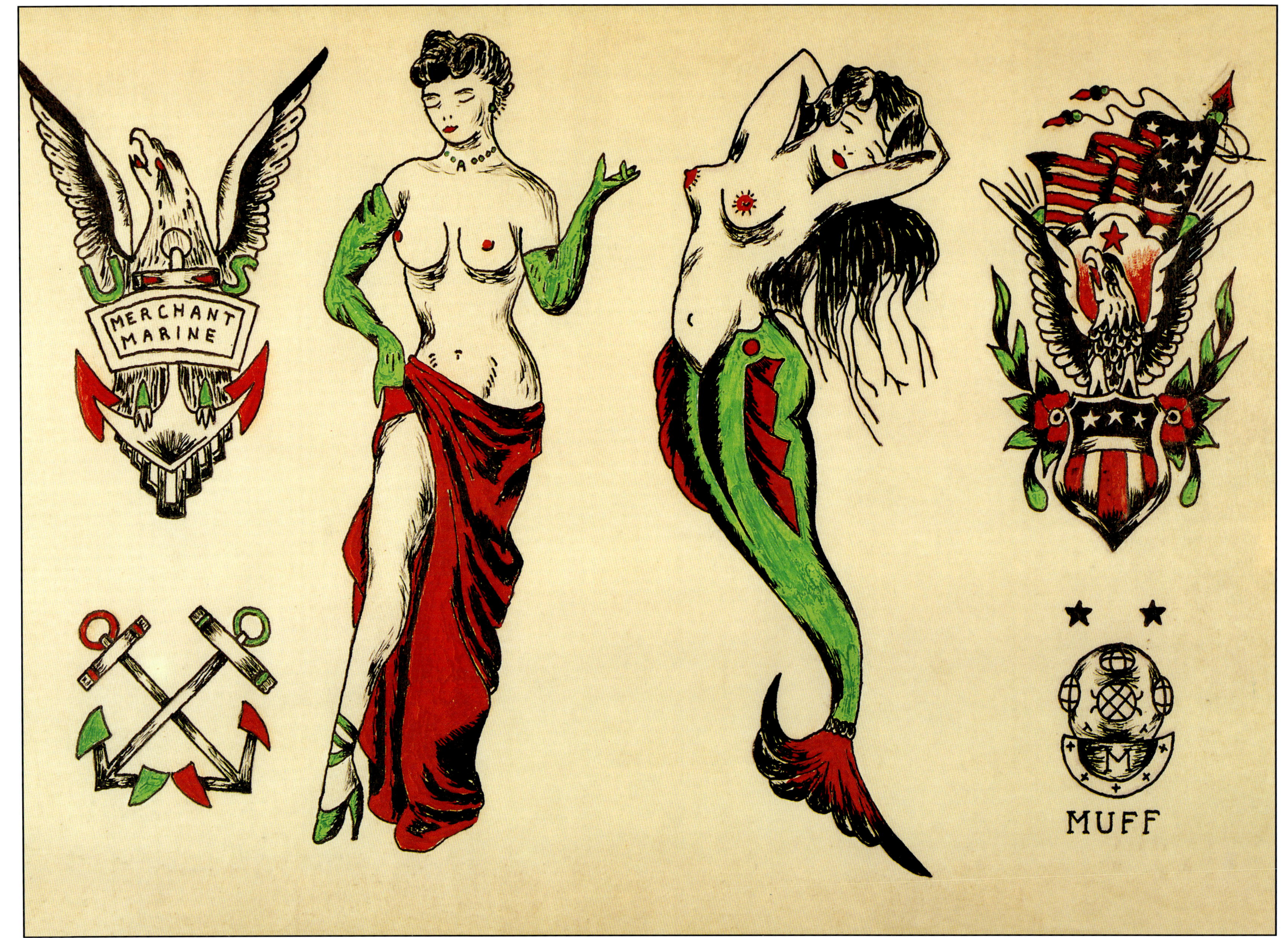
U S
MERCHANT
MARINE
M
MUFF

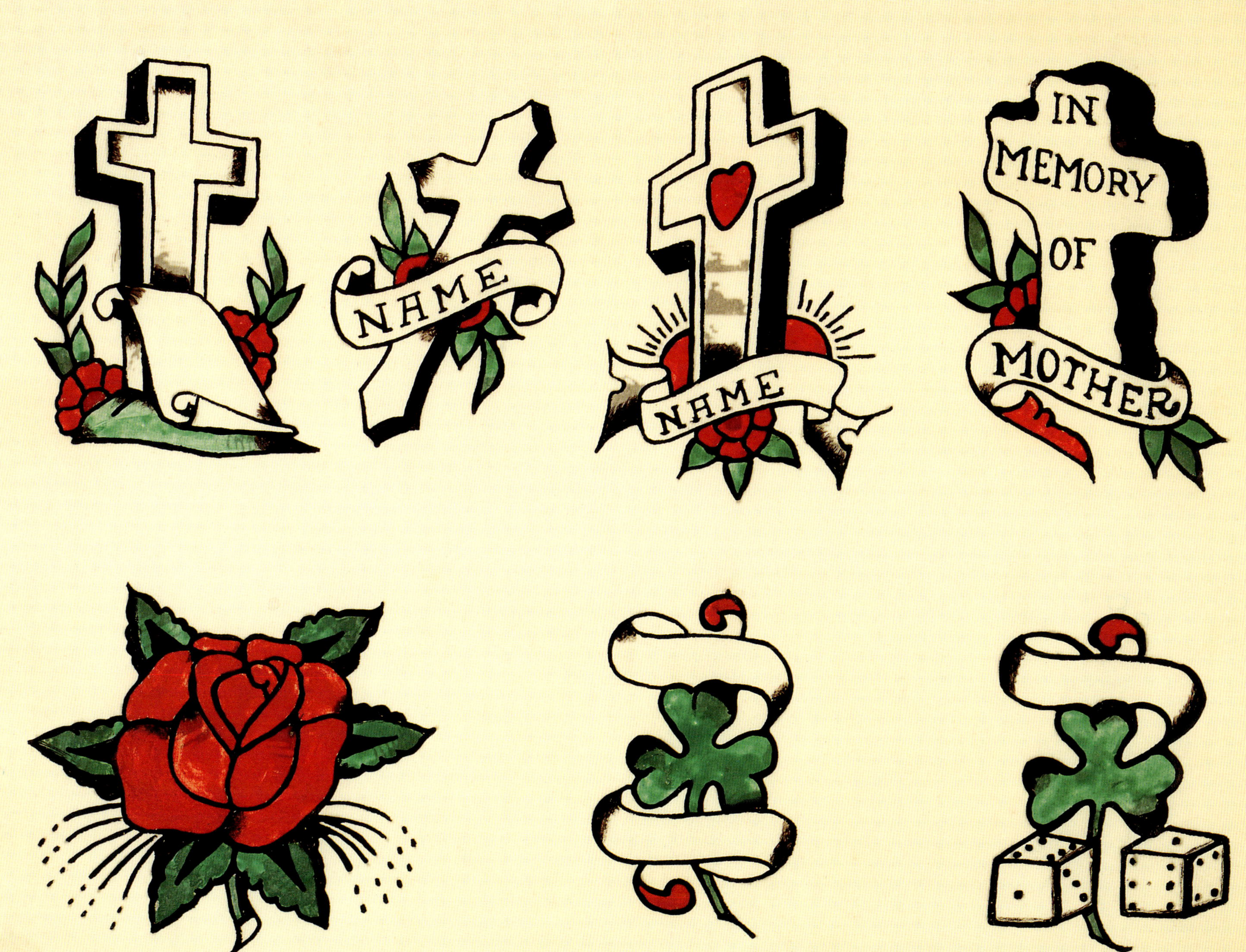
NAME
NAME
IN
MEMORY
OF
MOTHER

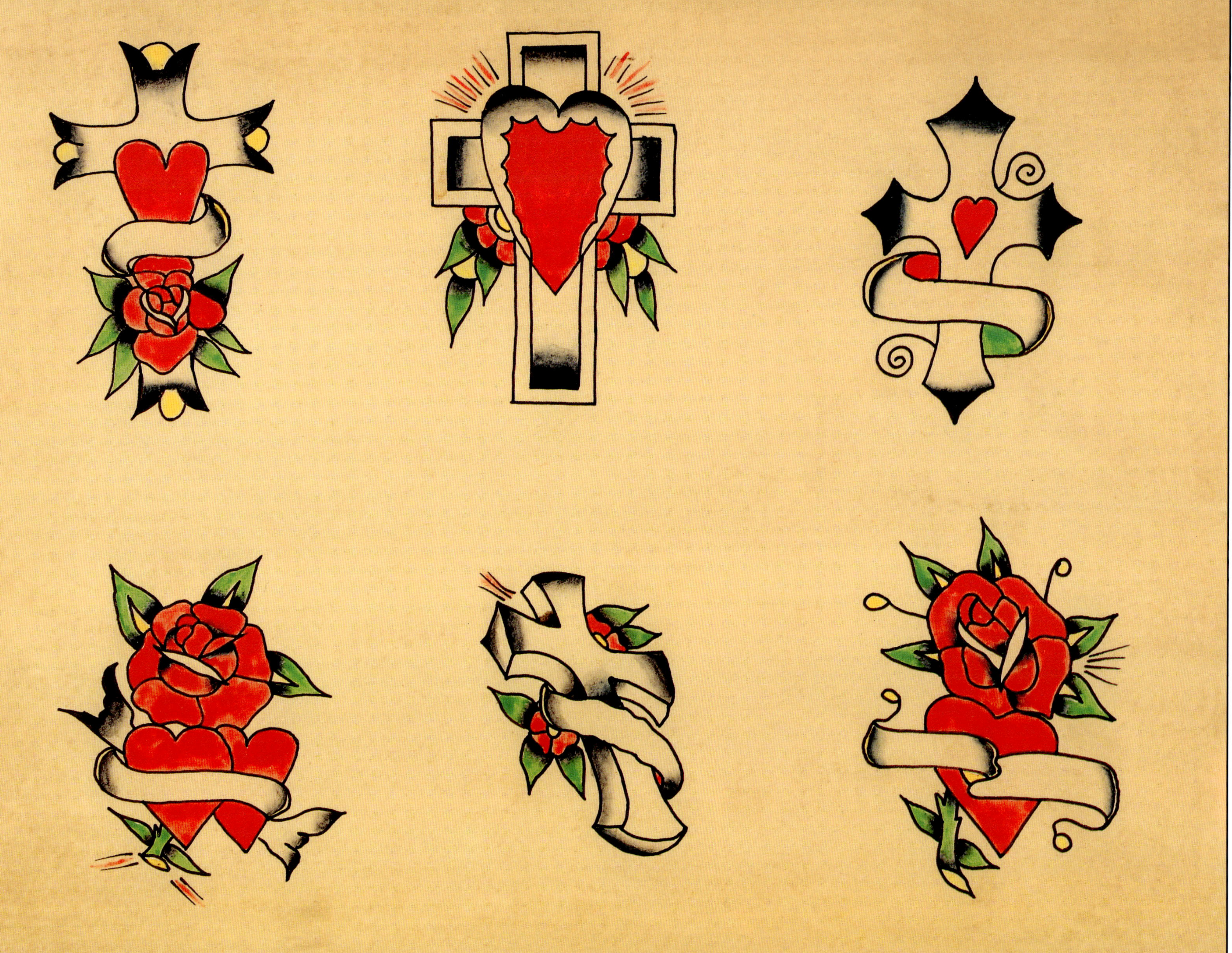

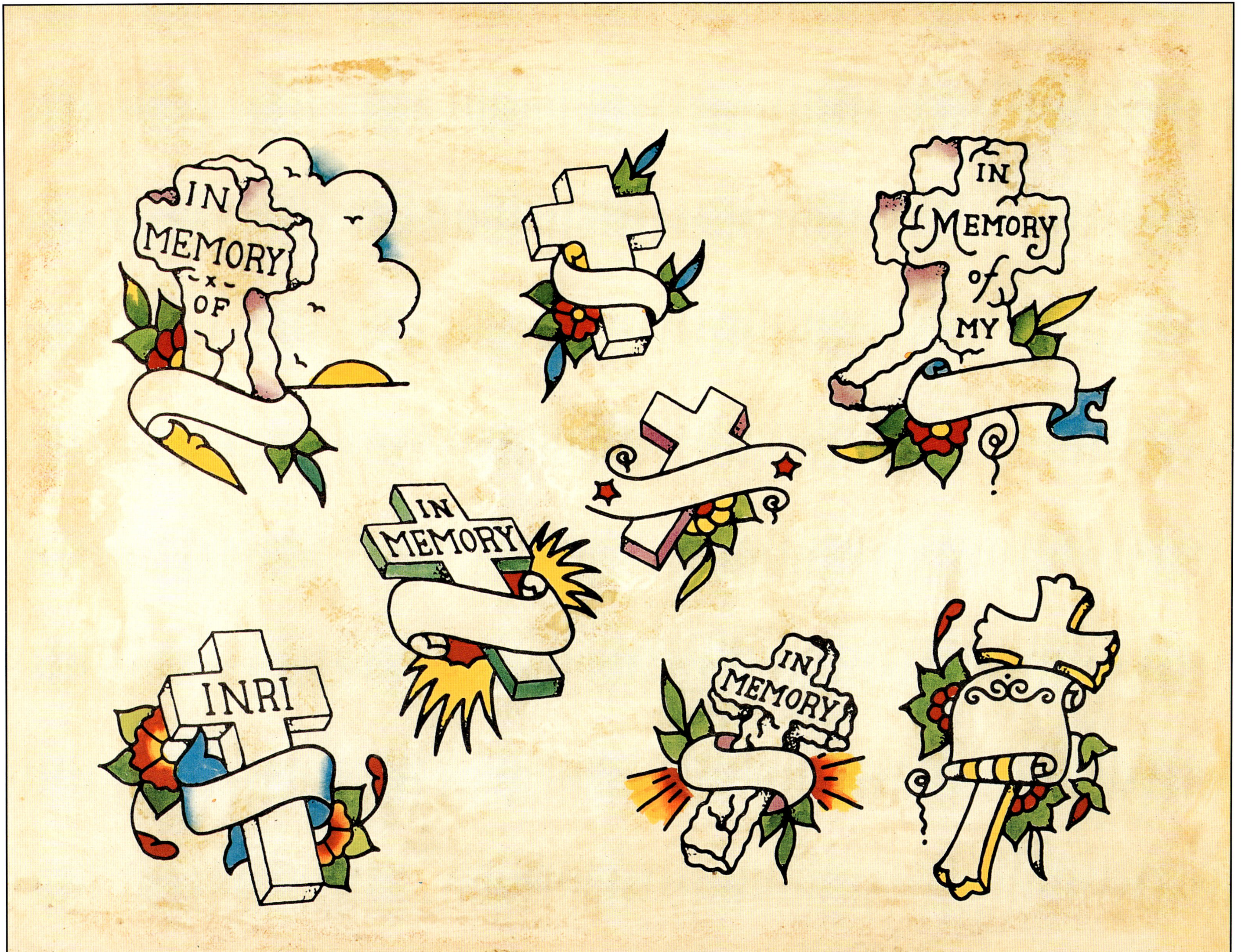
IN
MEMORY
OF
IN
MEMORY
of
MY
IN
MEMORY
INRI
IN
MEMORY

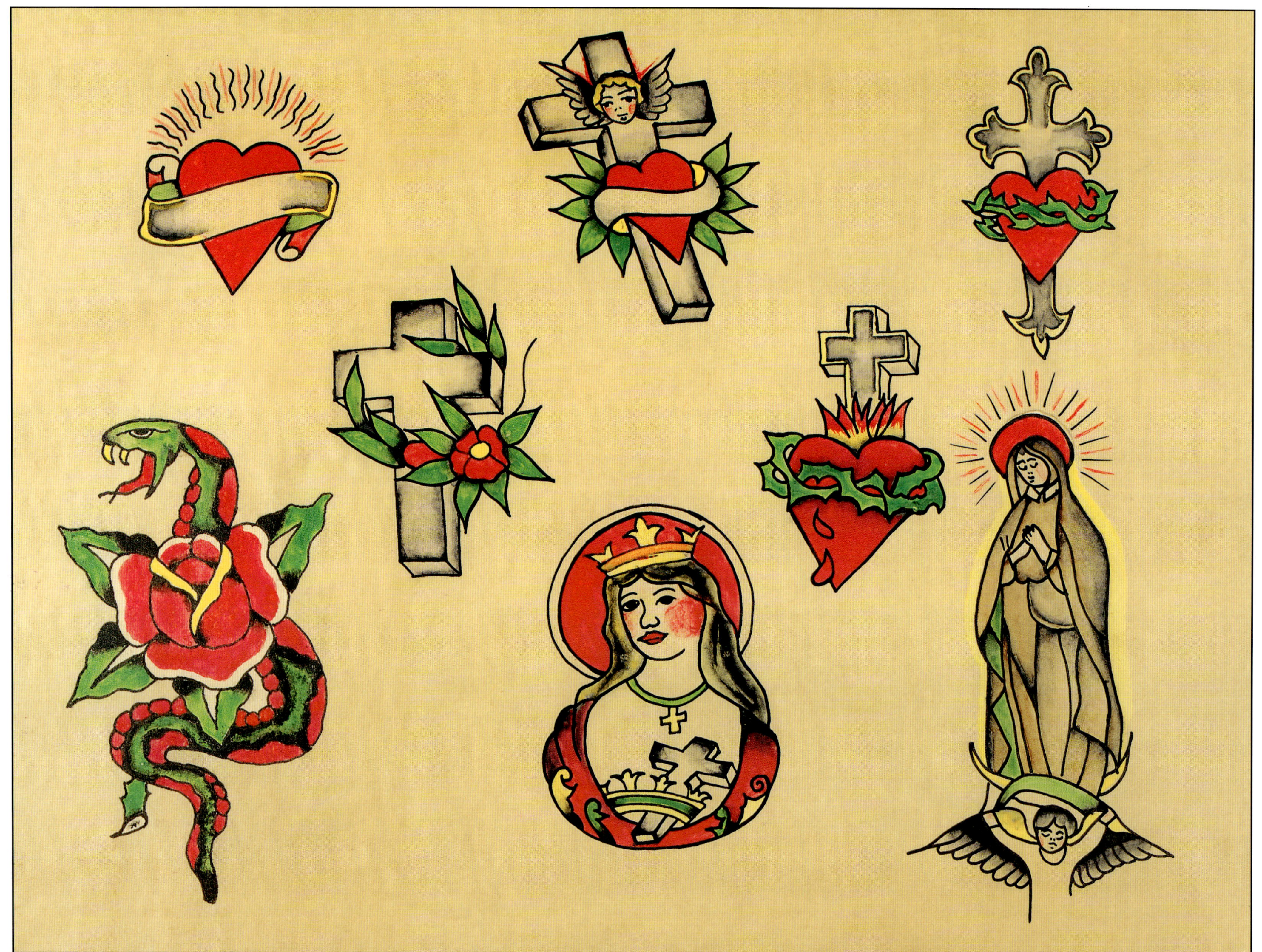

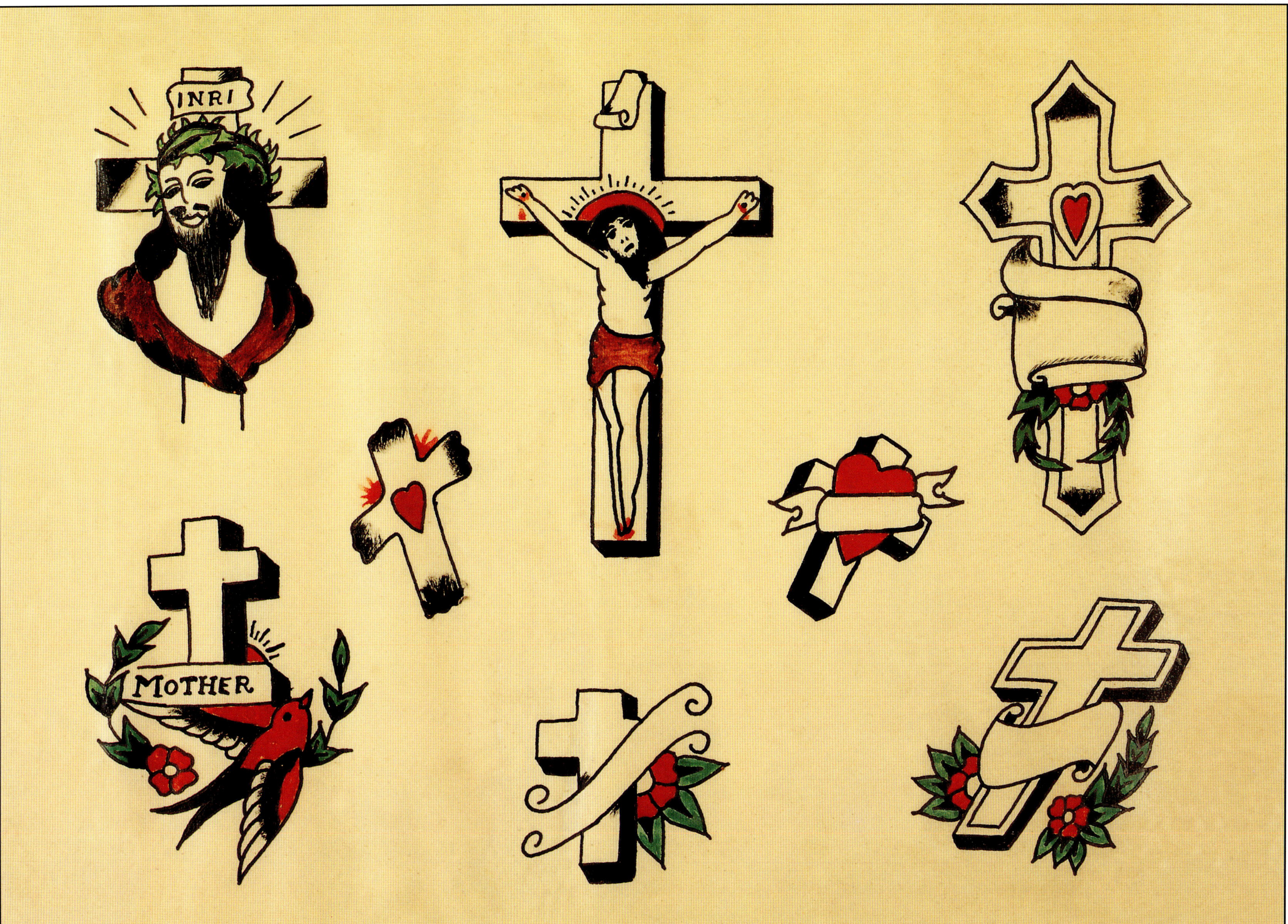
INRI
MOTHER

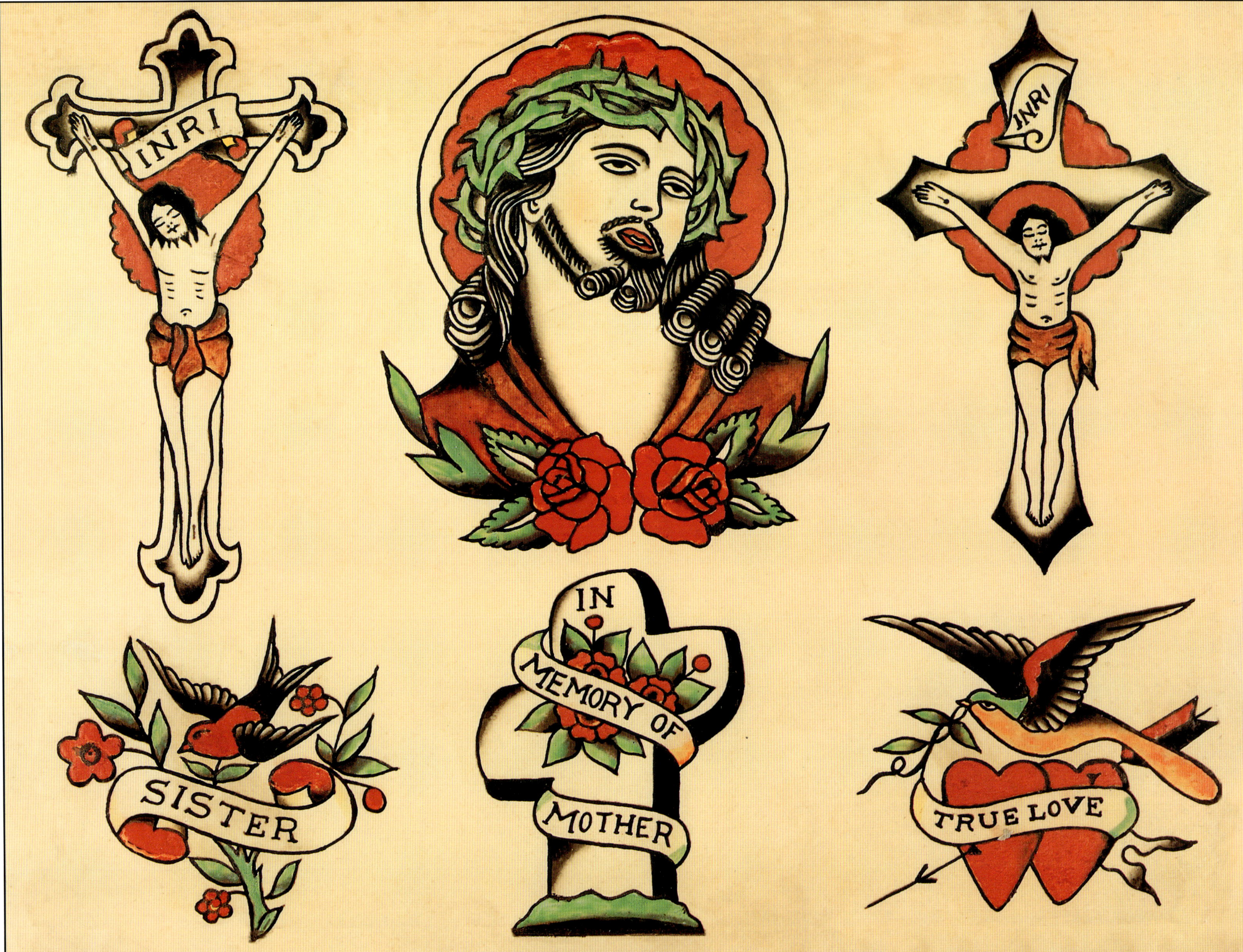
INRI
INRI
IN
MEMORY OF
MOTHER
SISTER
TRUE LOVE

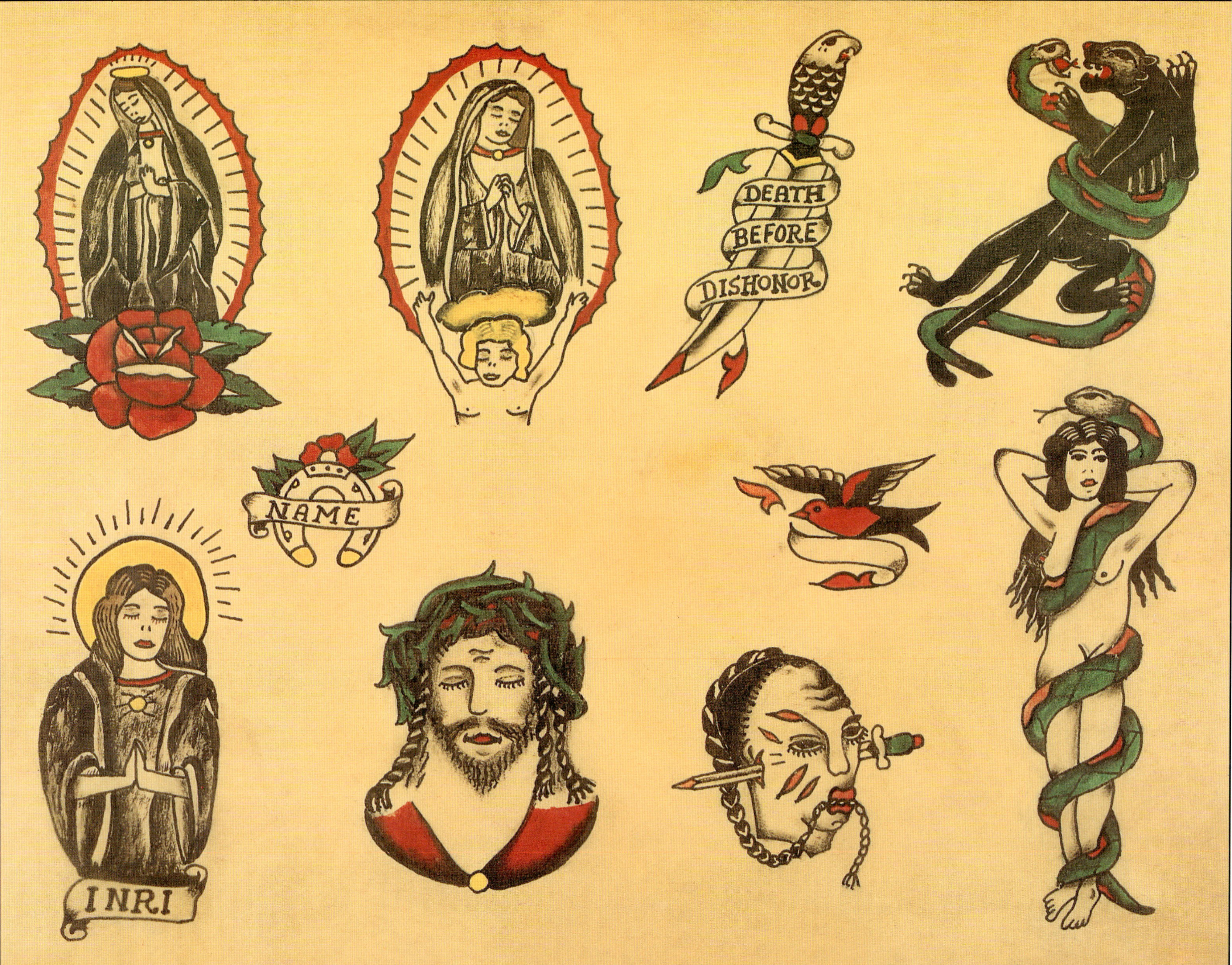
DEATH
BEFORE
DISHONOR
NAME
INRI

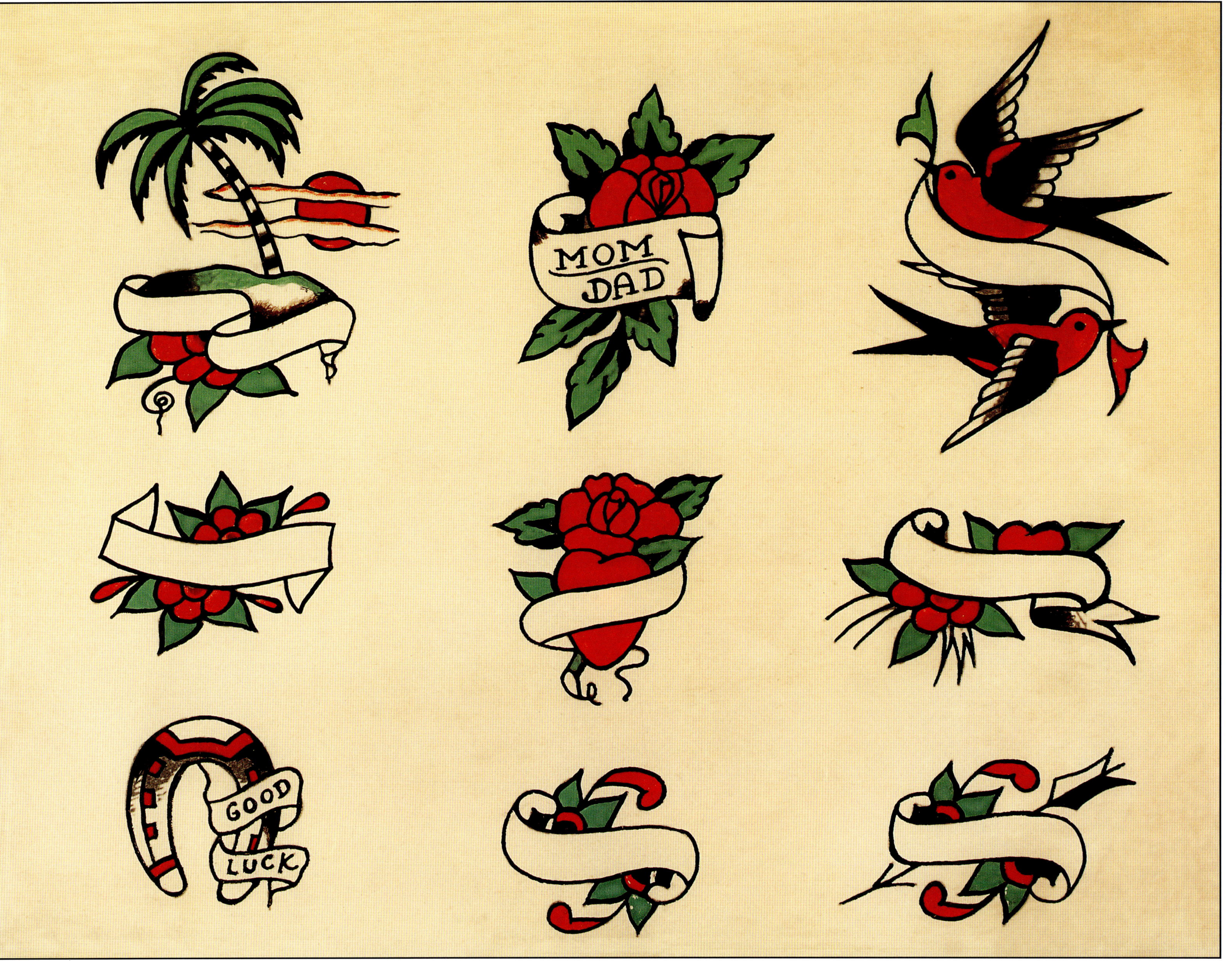
MOM
DAD
GOOD
LUCK

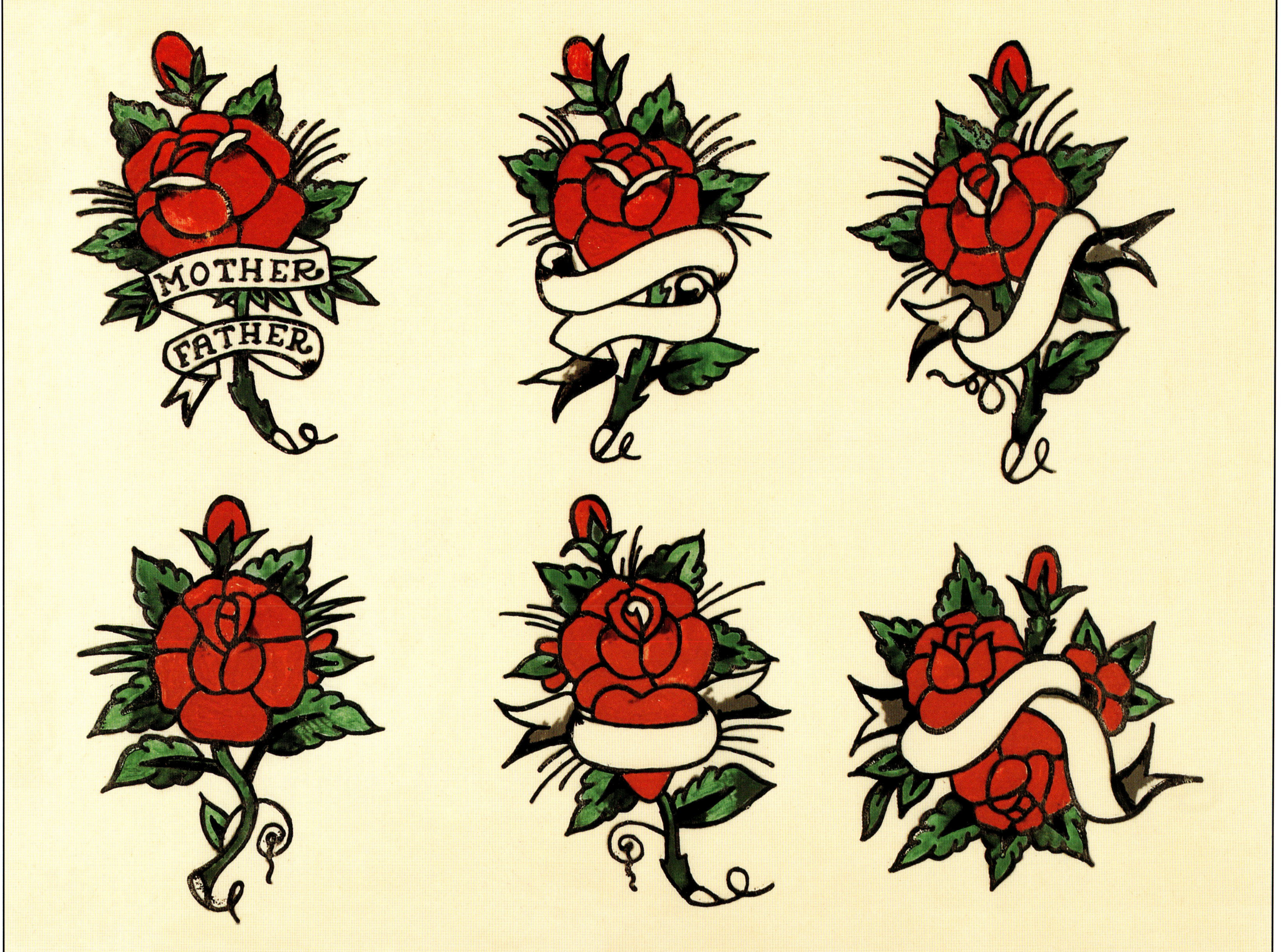
MOTHER
FATHER

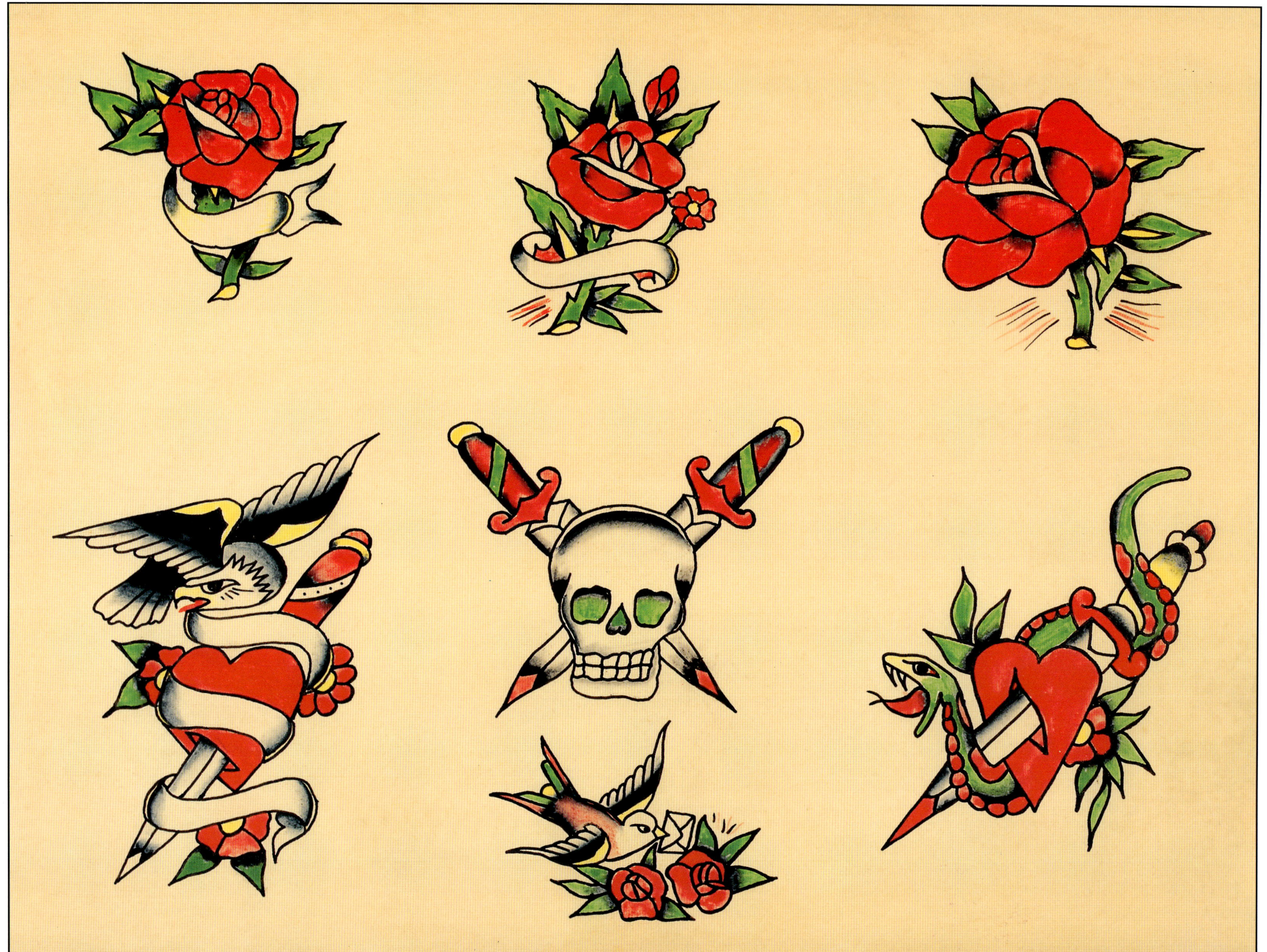

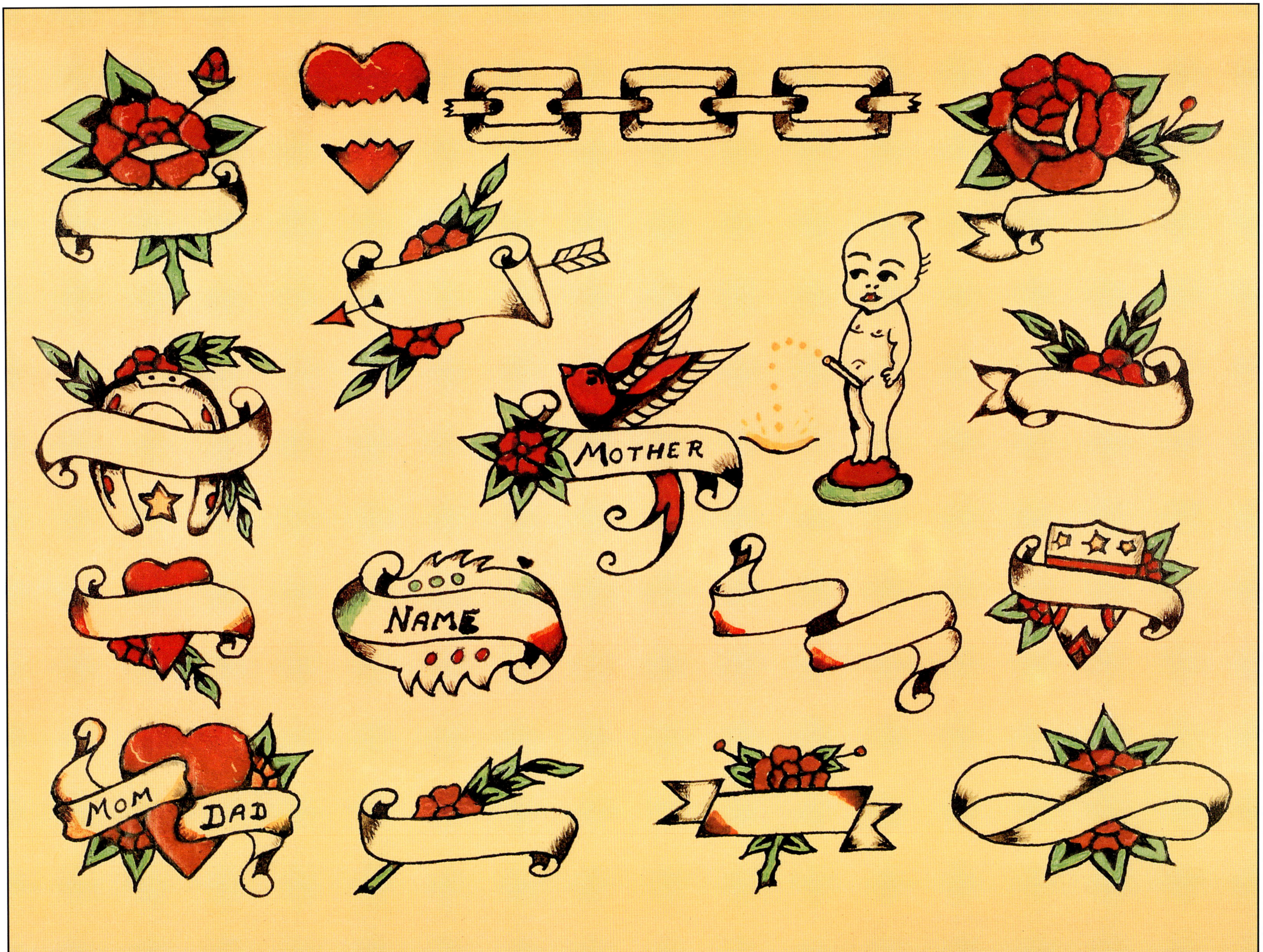
MOTHER
NAME
MOM
DAD

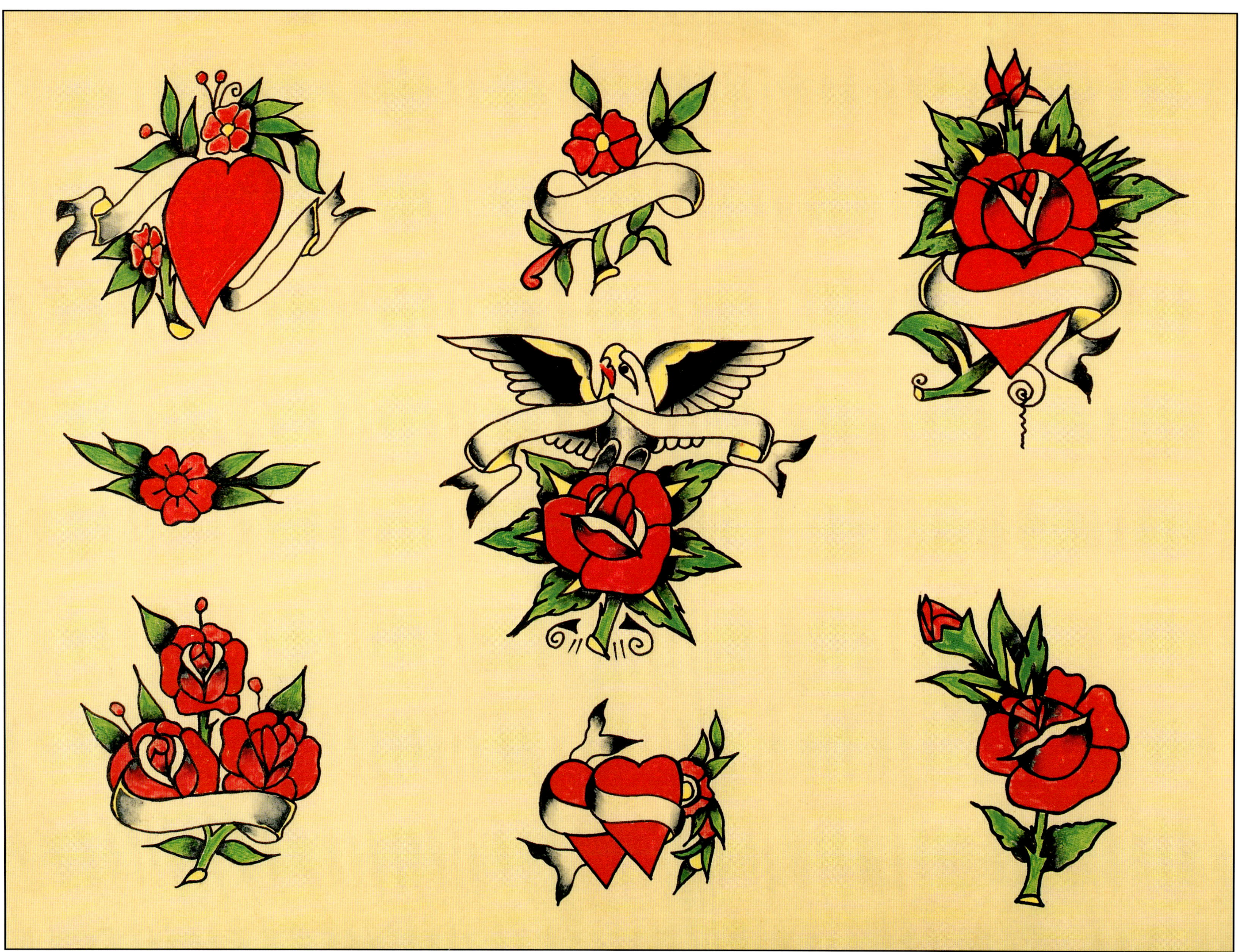

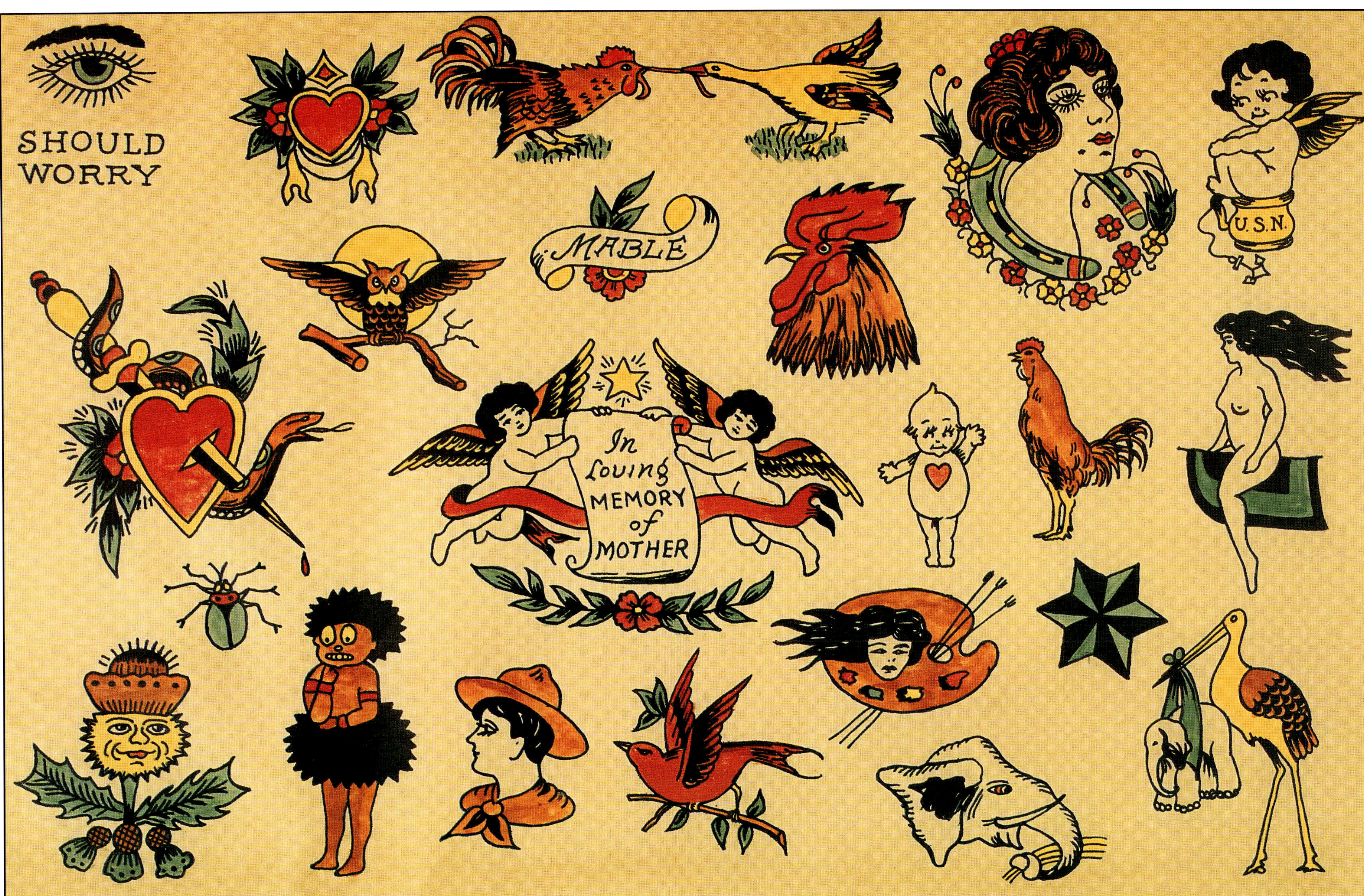
SHOULD
WORRY
MABLE
U.S.N.
In Loving MEMORY of MOTHER

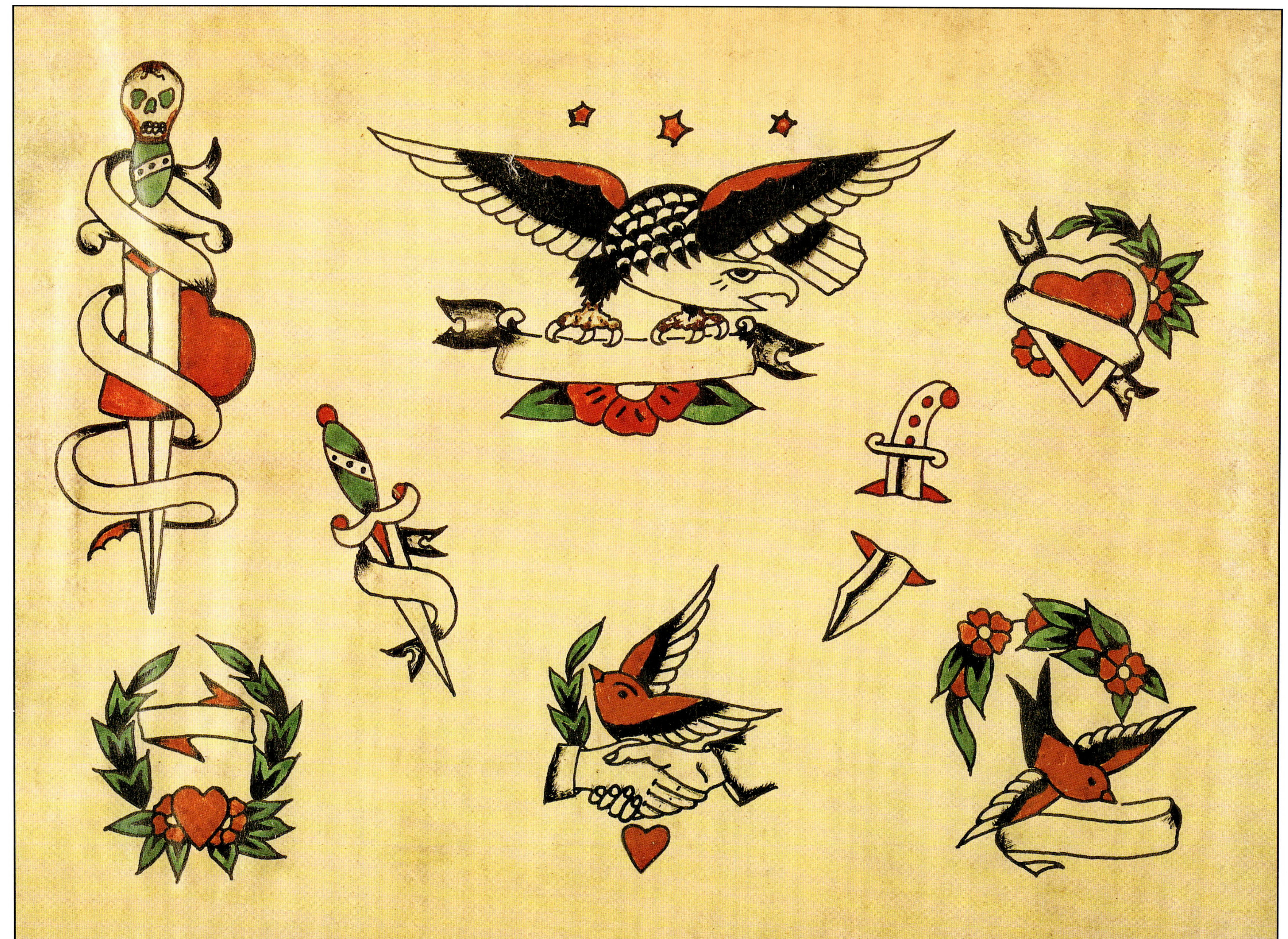

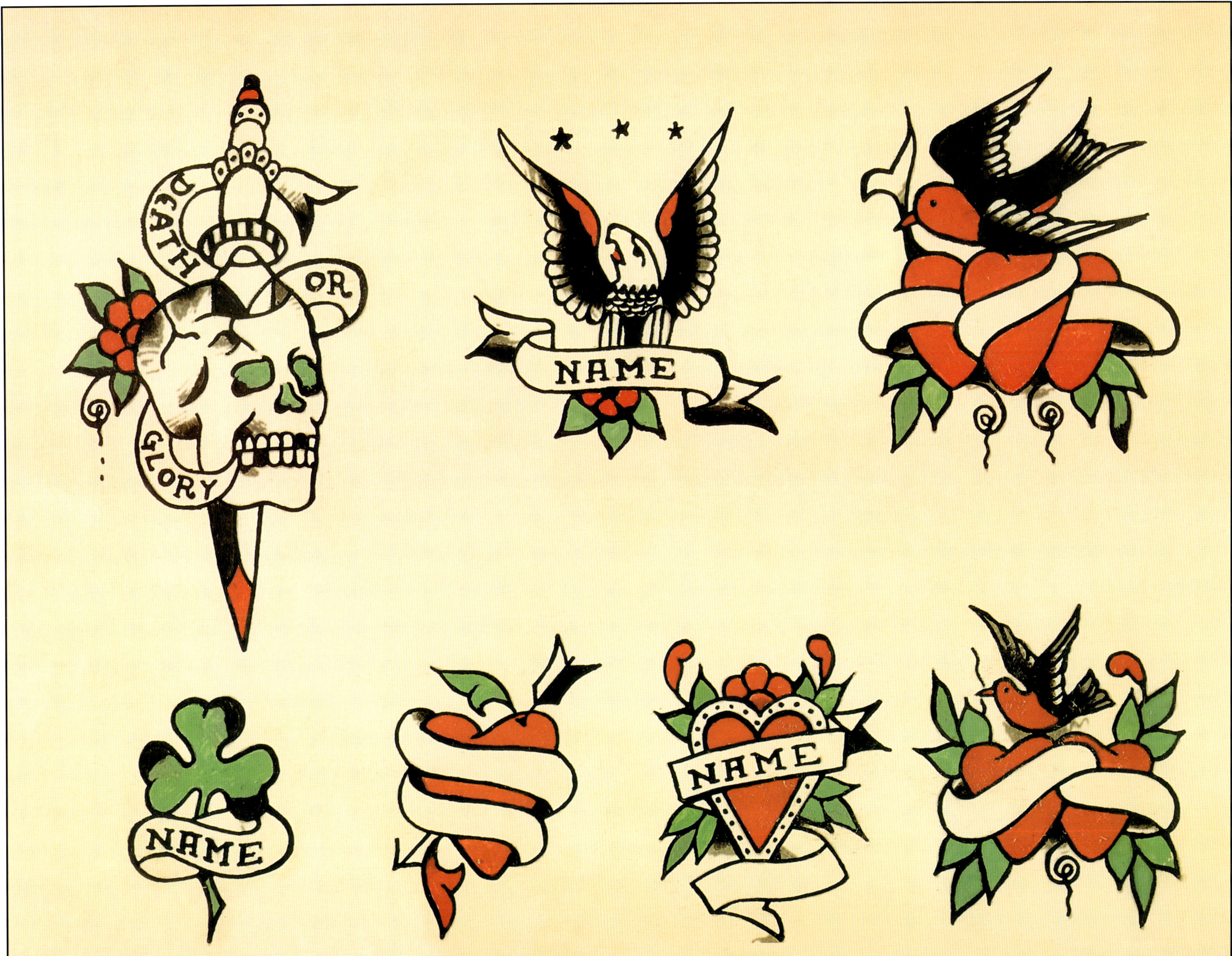
DEATH
OR
GLORY
NAME
NAME
NAME

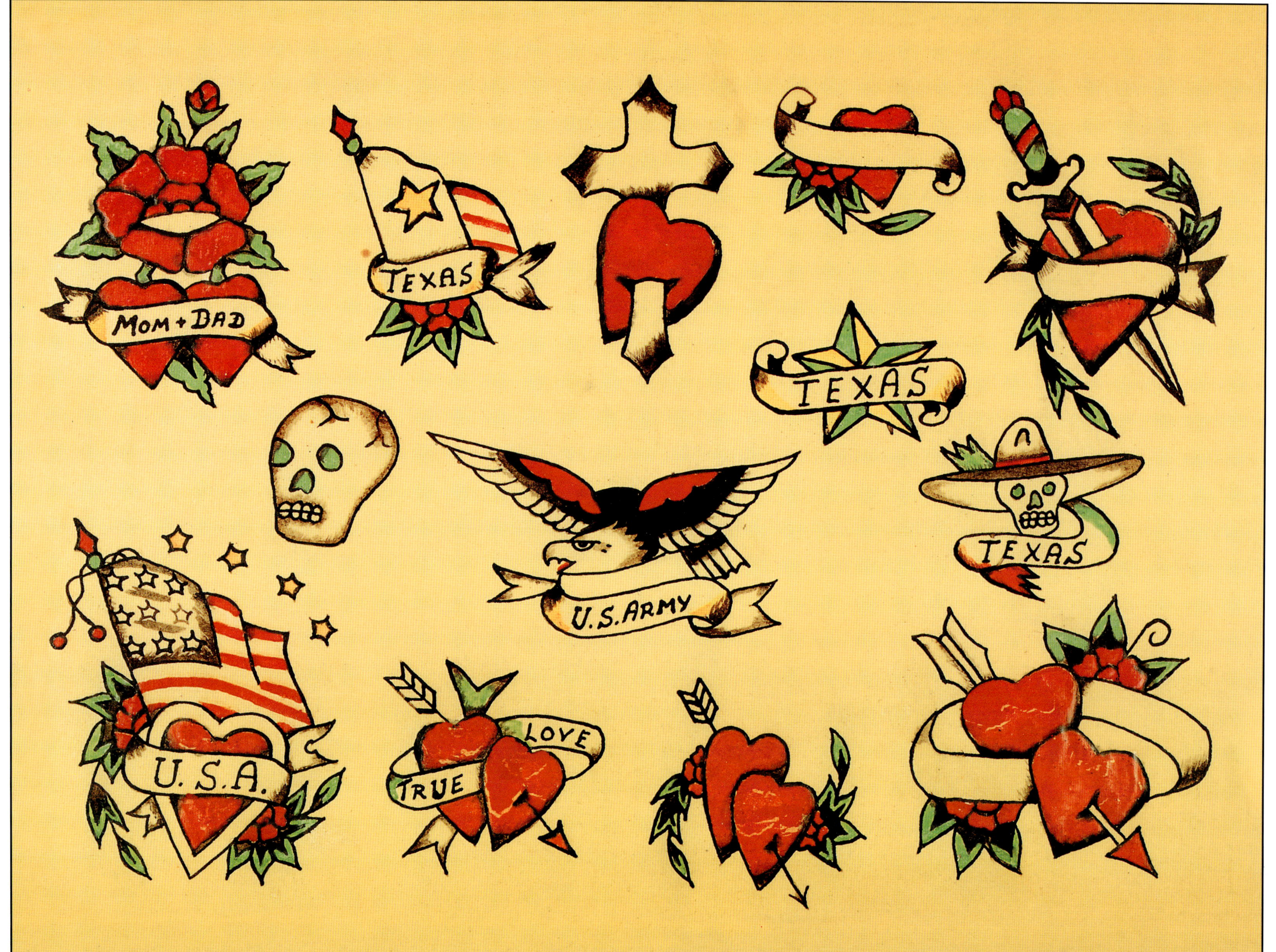
MOM + DAD
TEXAS
TEXAS
TEXAS
U.S. ARMY
U.S.A.
LOVE
TRUE

NAME
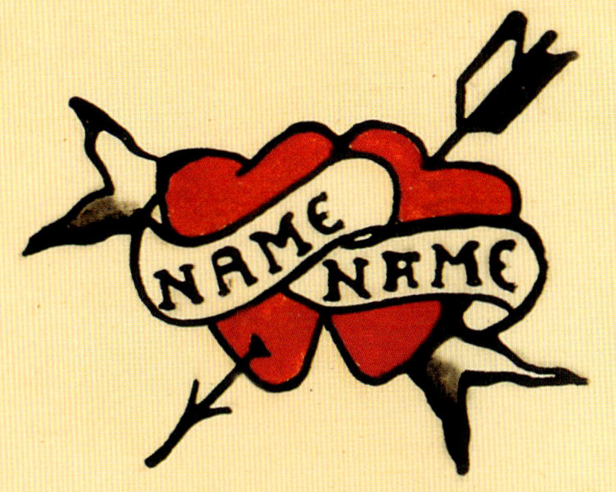
NAME
NAME
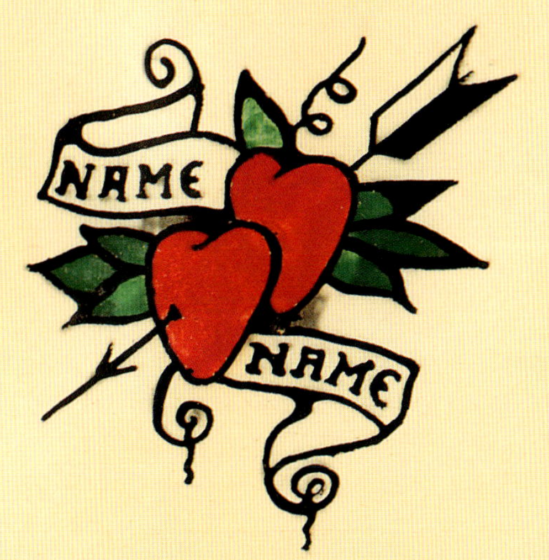
NAME
NAME
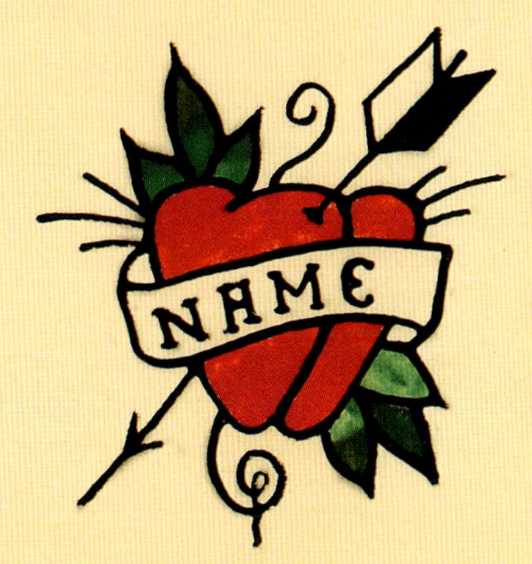
NAME
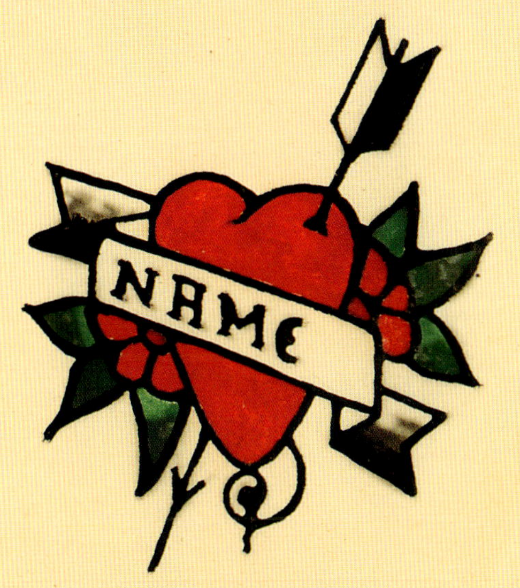
NAME
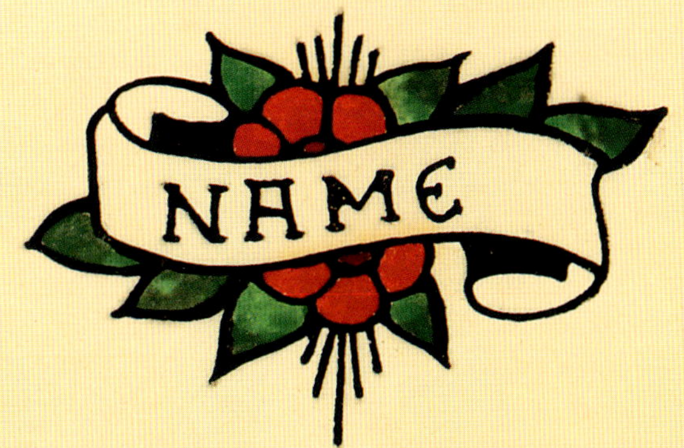
NAME
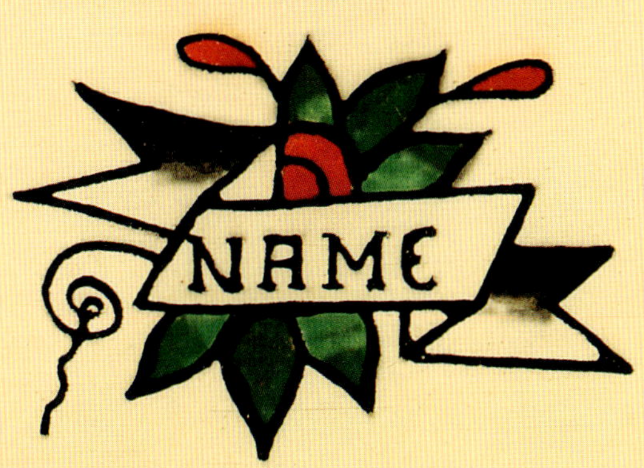
NAME

NAME

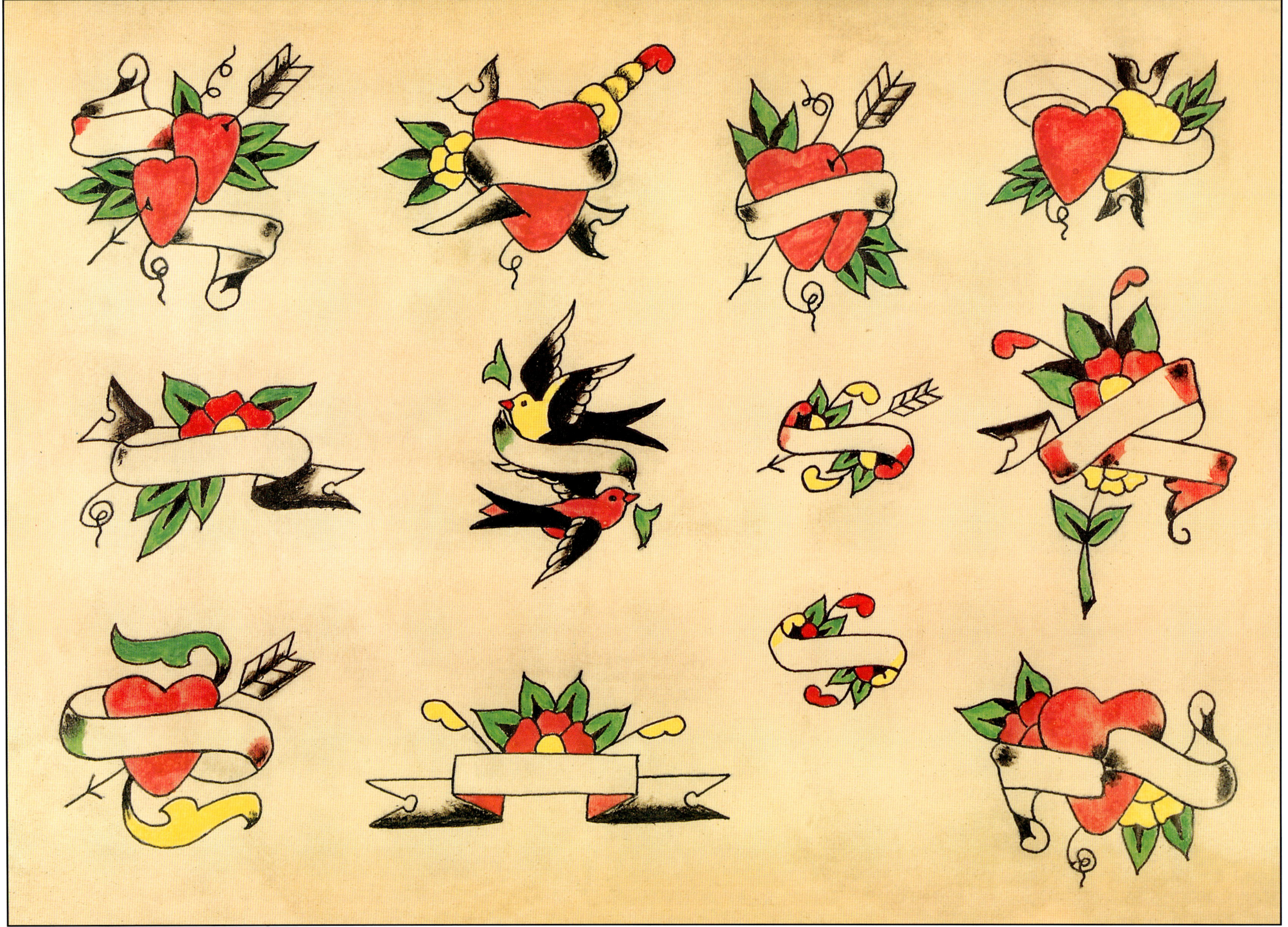

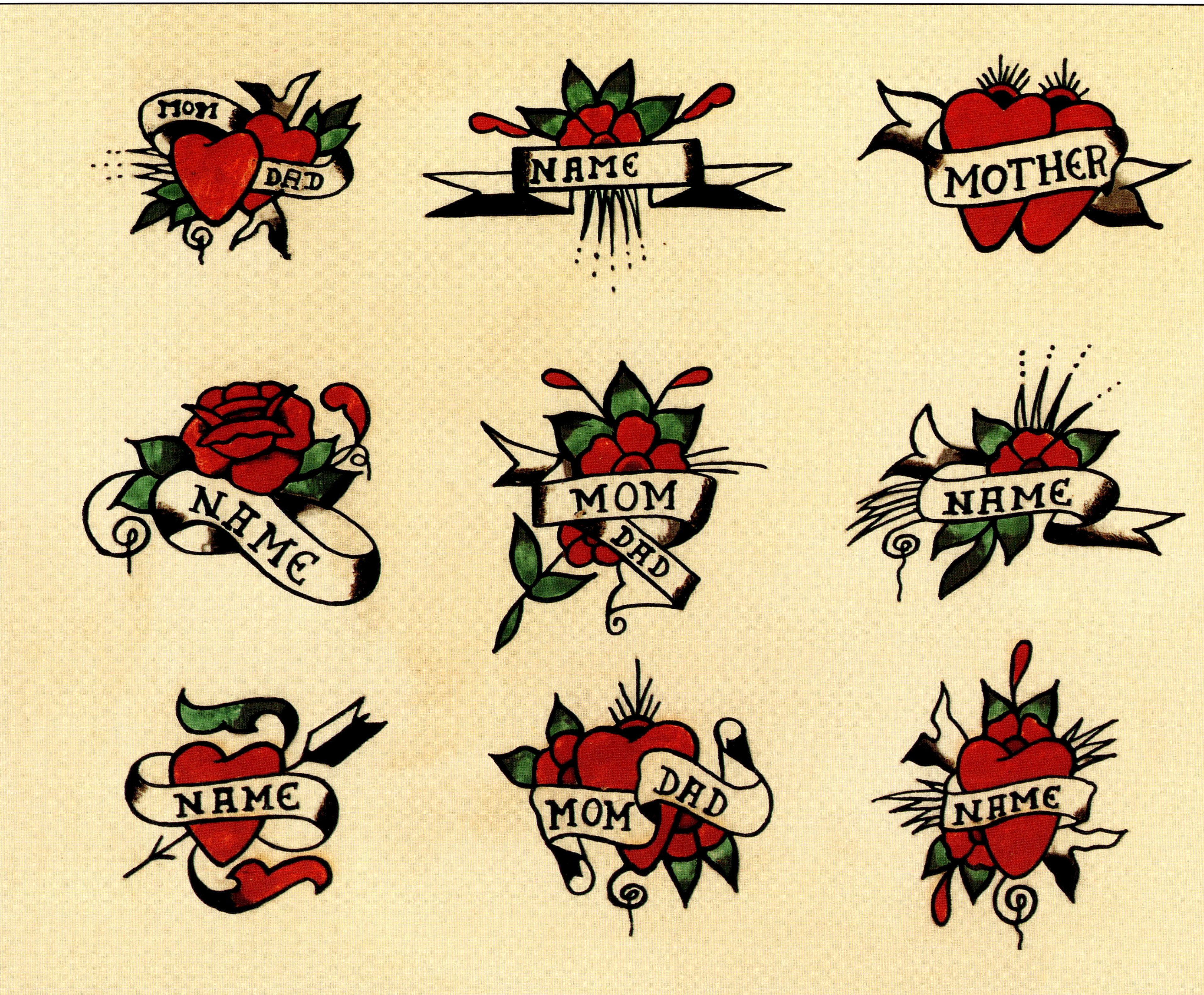
MOM
DAD
NAME
MOTHER
NAME
MOM
DAD
NAME
NAME
MOM
DAD
NAME

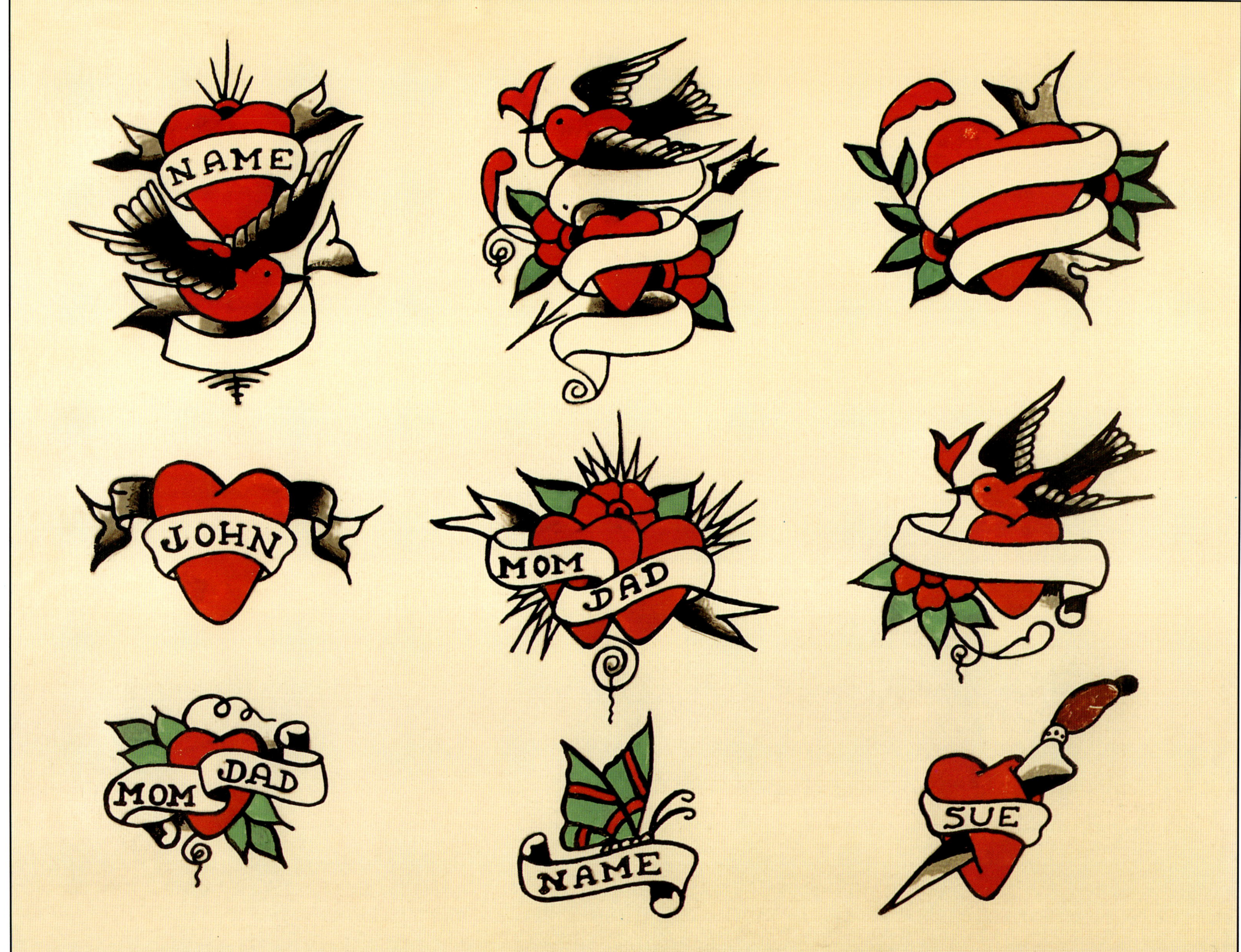
NAME
JOHN
MOM
DAD
MOM
DAD
NAME
SUE

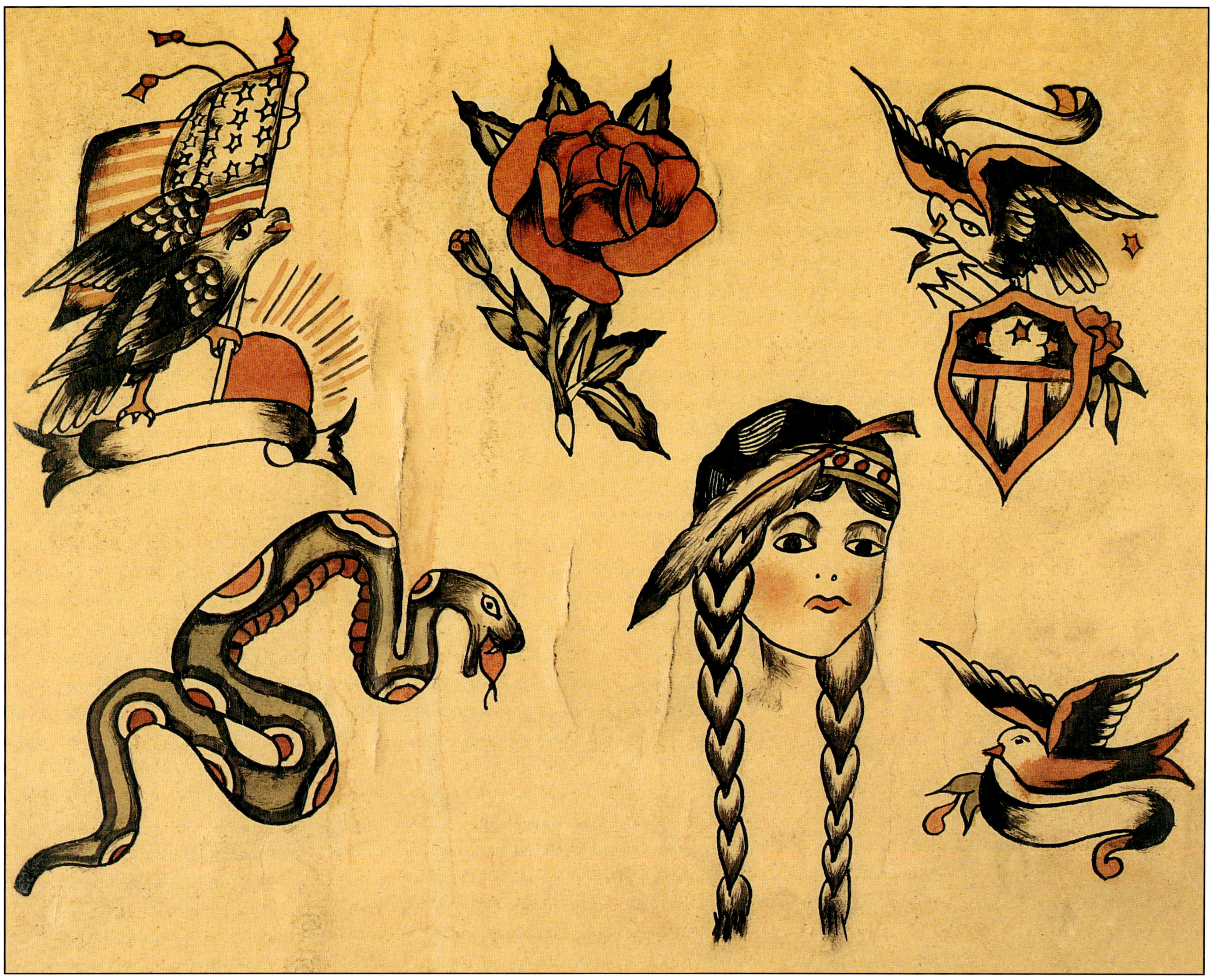

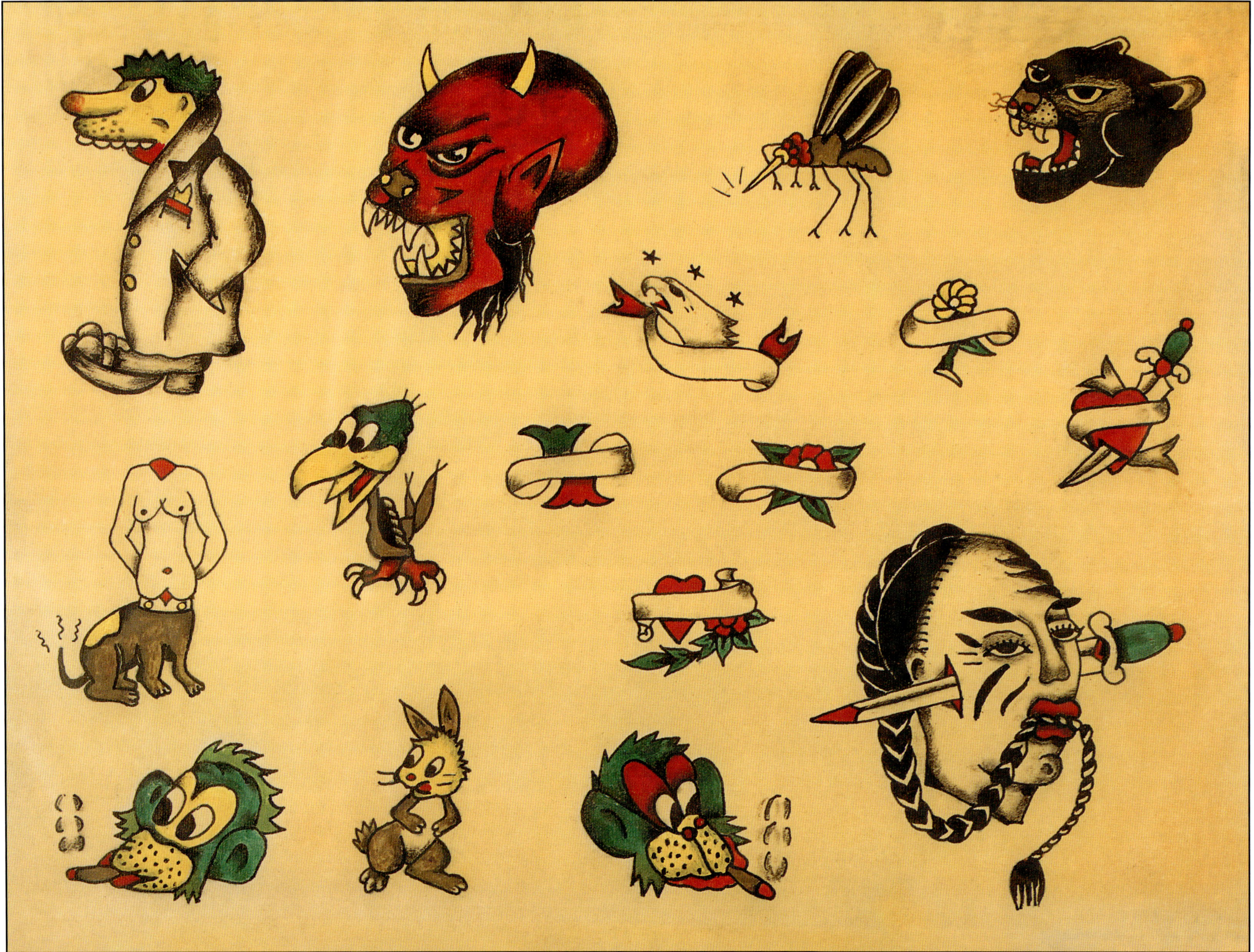

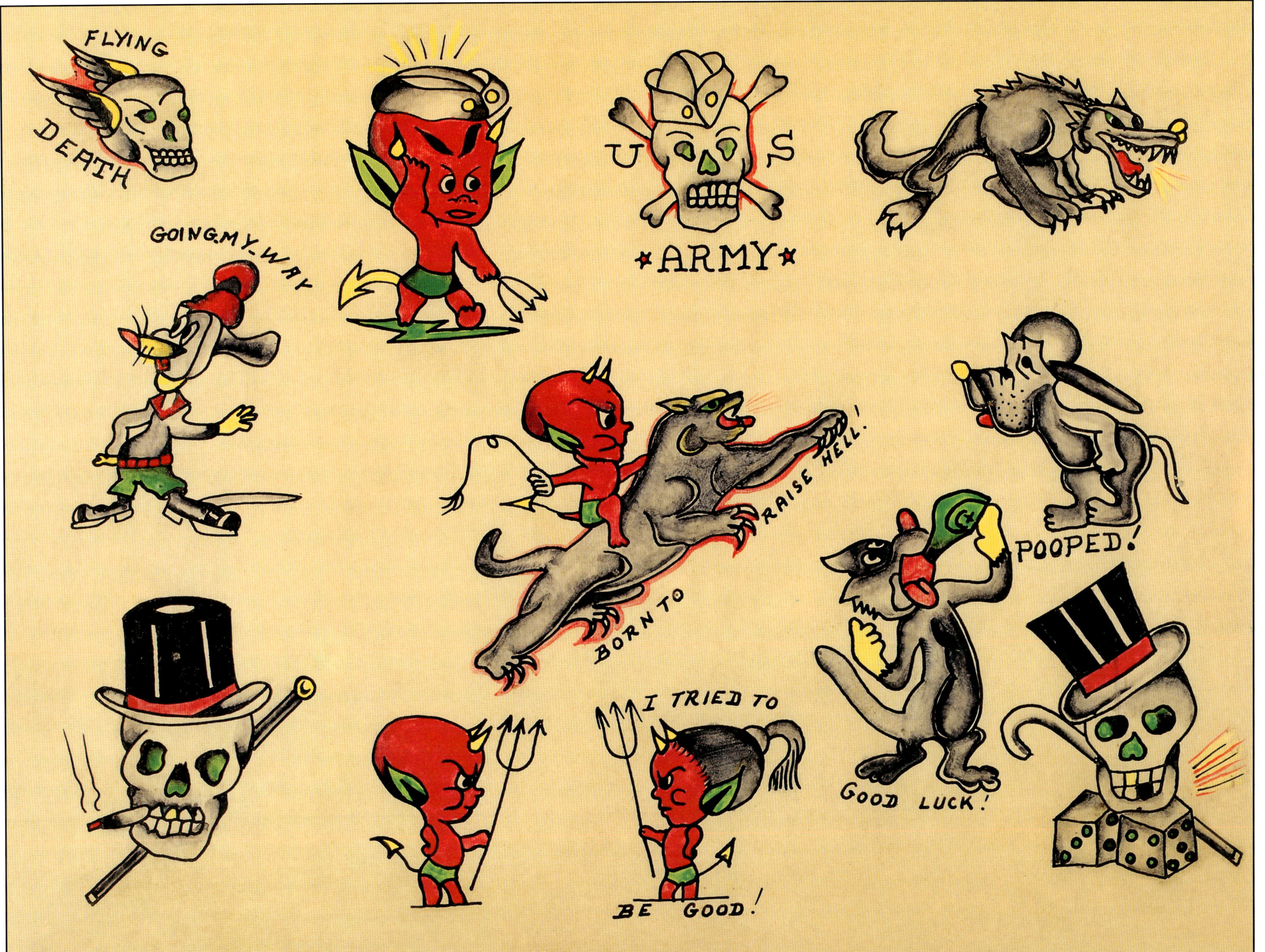
FLYING
DEATH
U S
ARMY
GOING MY WAY
BORN TO
RAISE HELL!
POOPED!
GOOD LUCK!
I TRIED TO
BE GOOD!

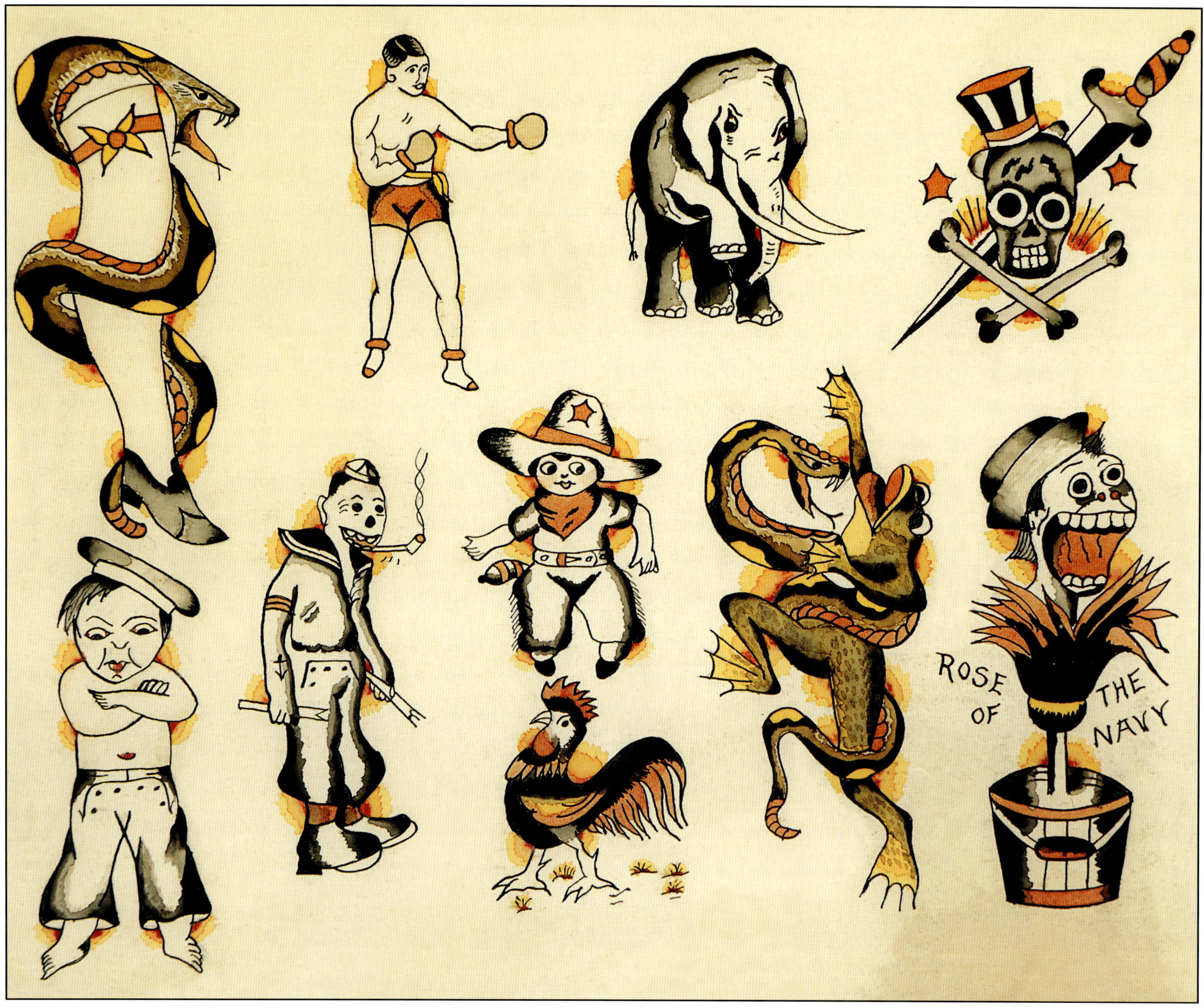
ROSE OF THE NAVY

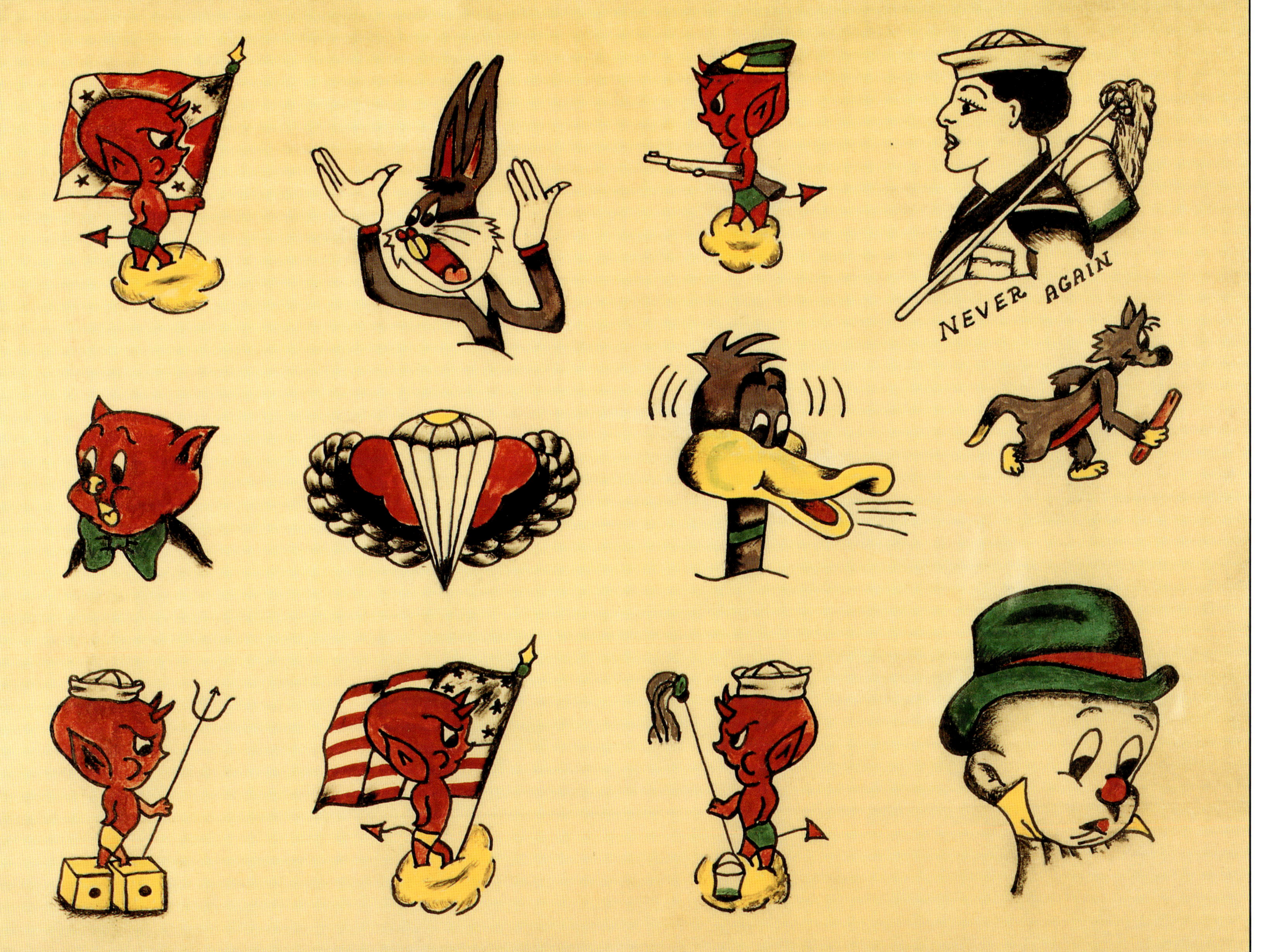
NEVER AGAIN

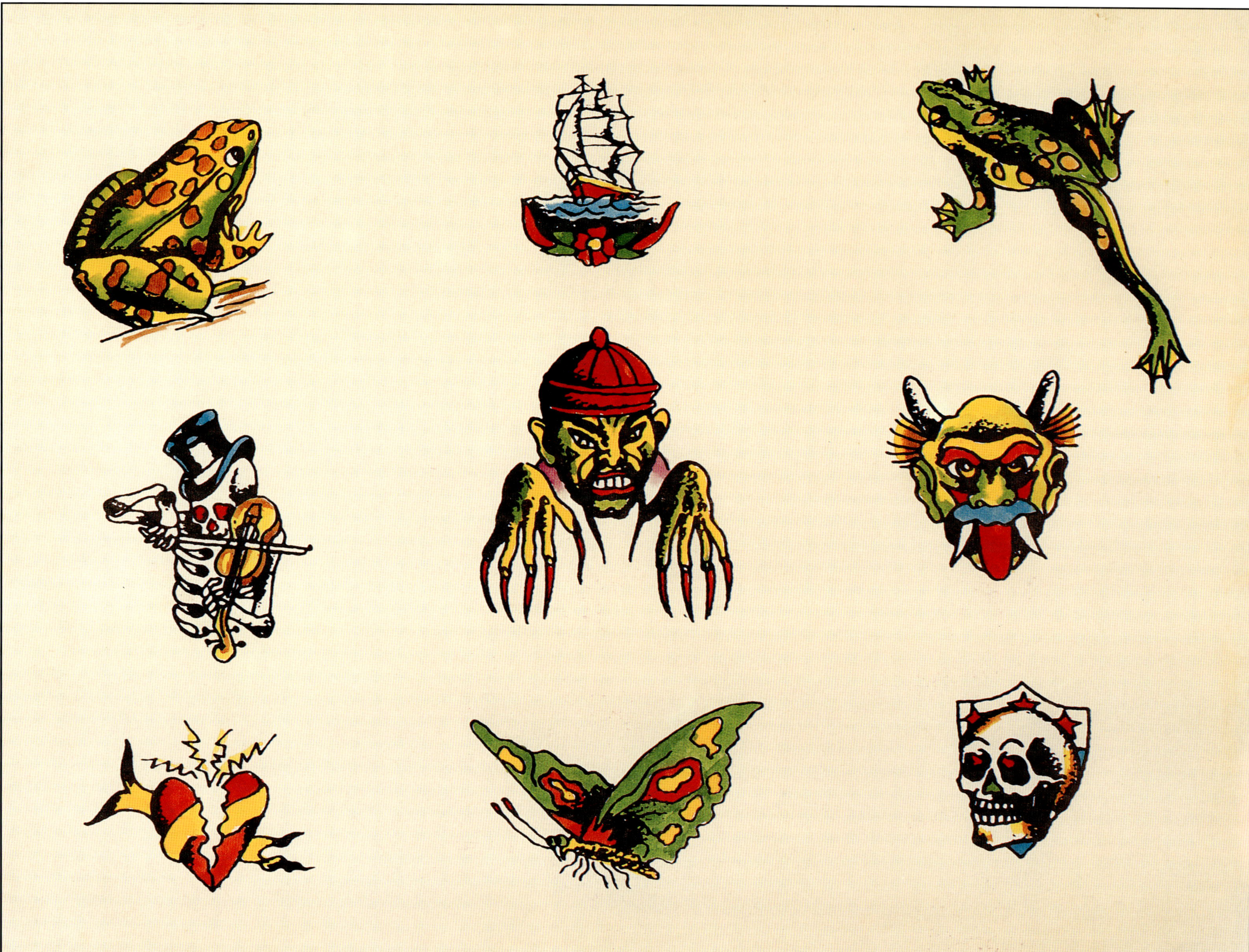

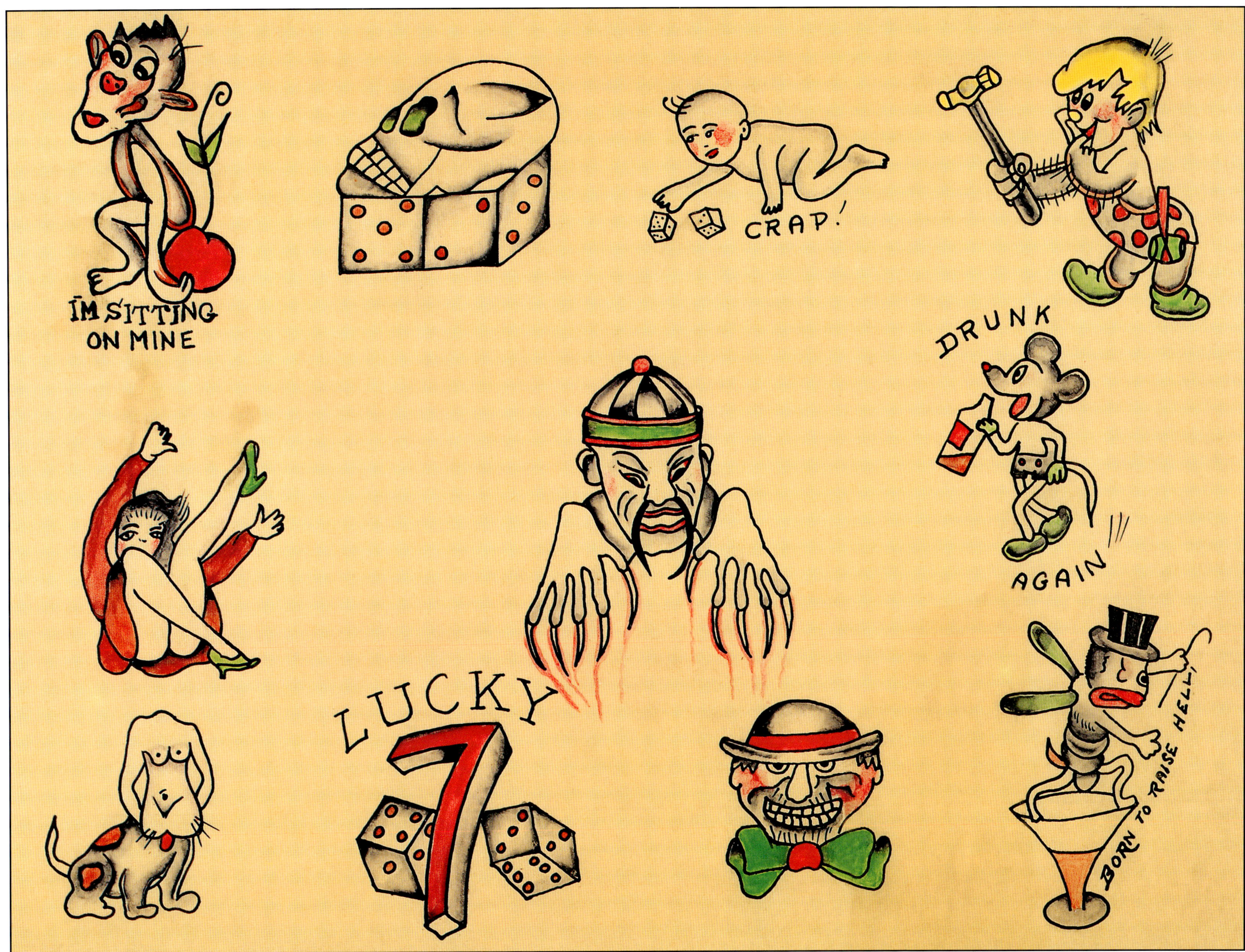
I'M SITTING
ON MINE
CRAP!
DRUNK
AGAIN
LUCKY
BORN TO RAISE HELL!

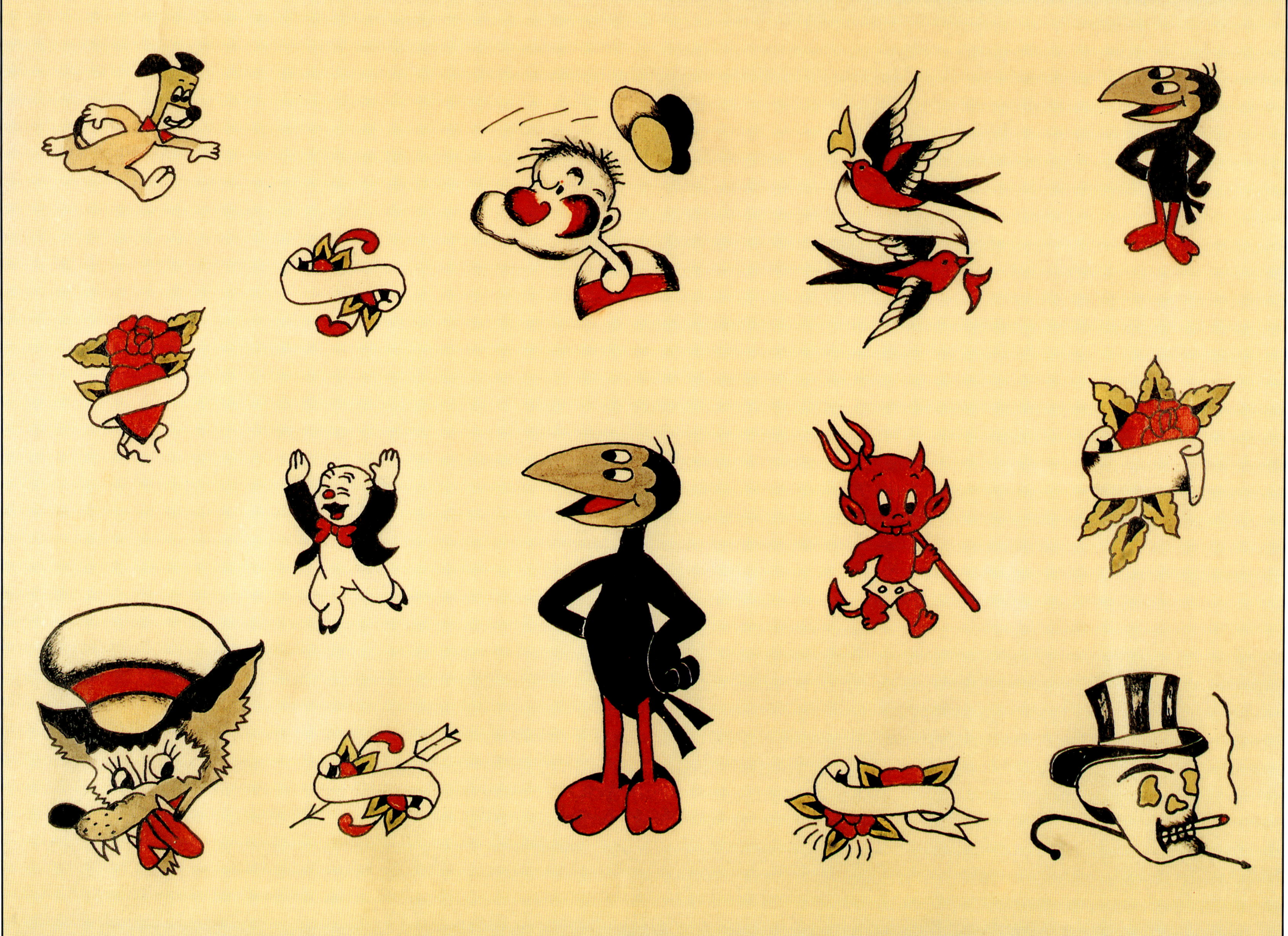

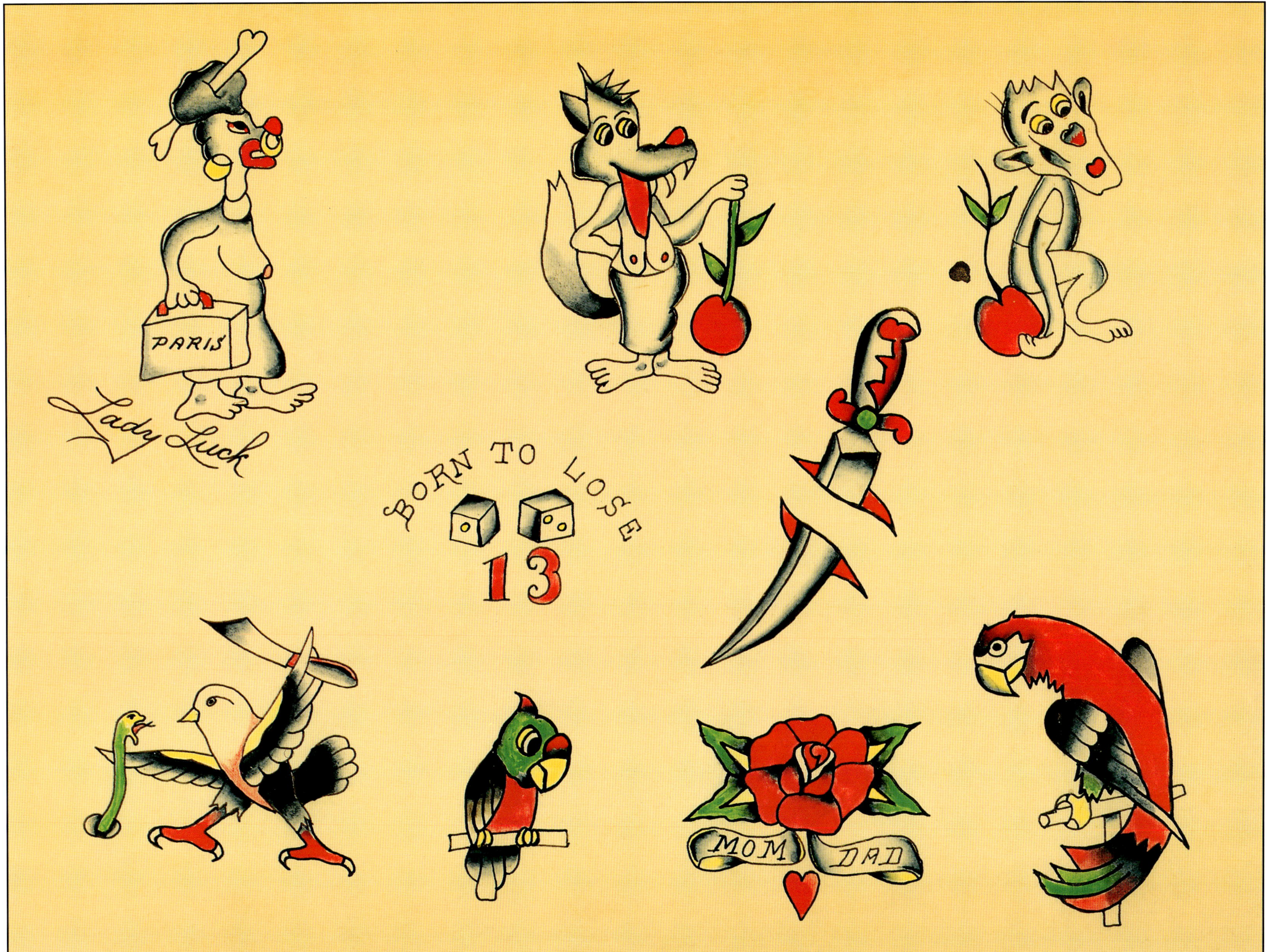

PARIS
Lady Luck
BORN TO LOSE
13
MOM
DAD

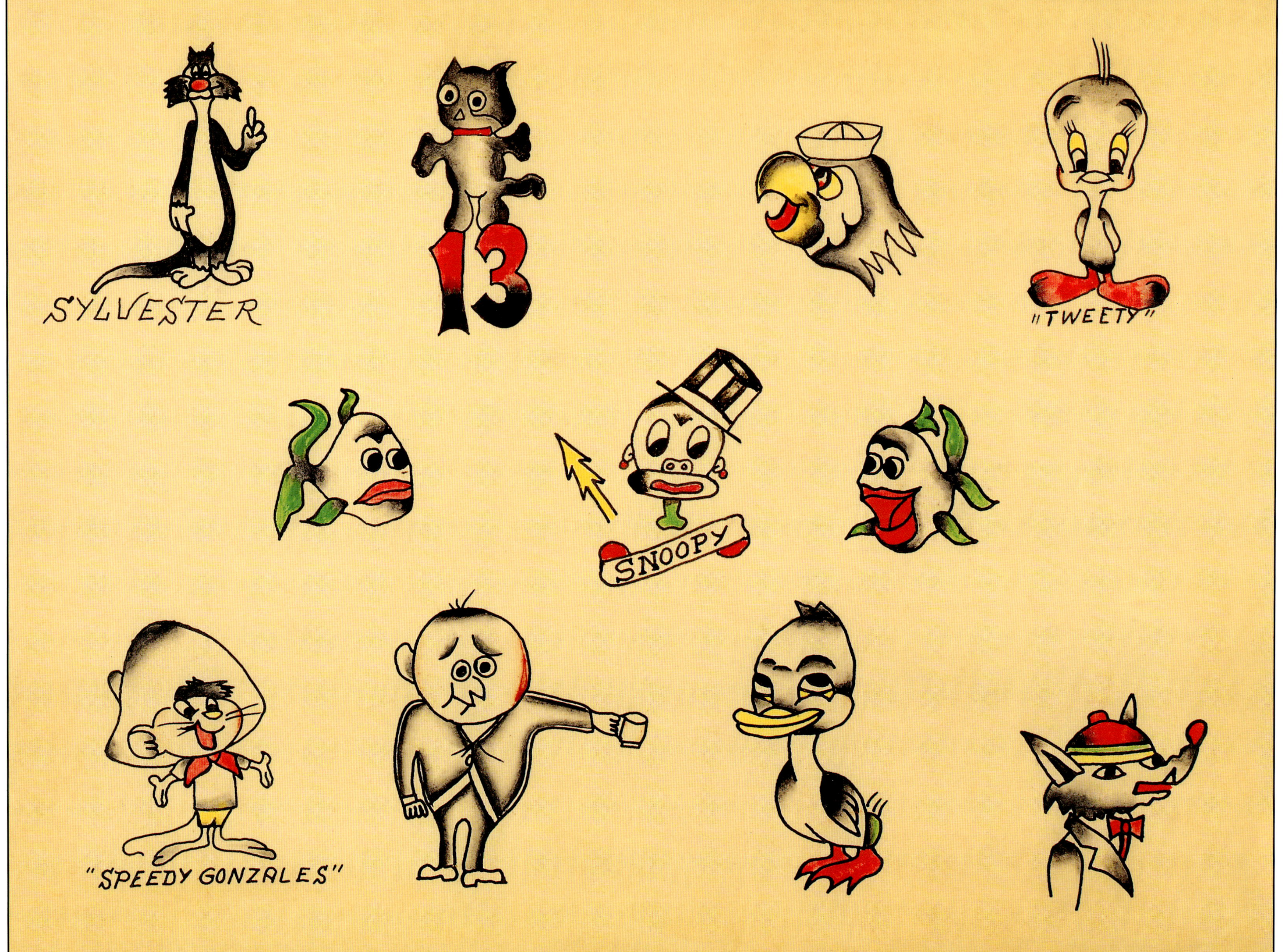
SYLVESTER
13
"TWEETY"
SNOOPY
"SPEEDY GONZALES"

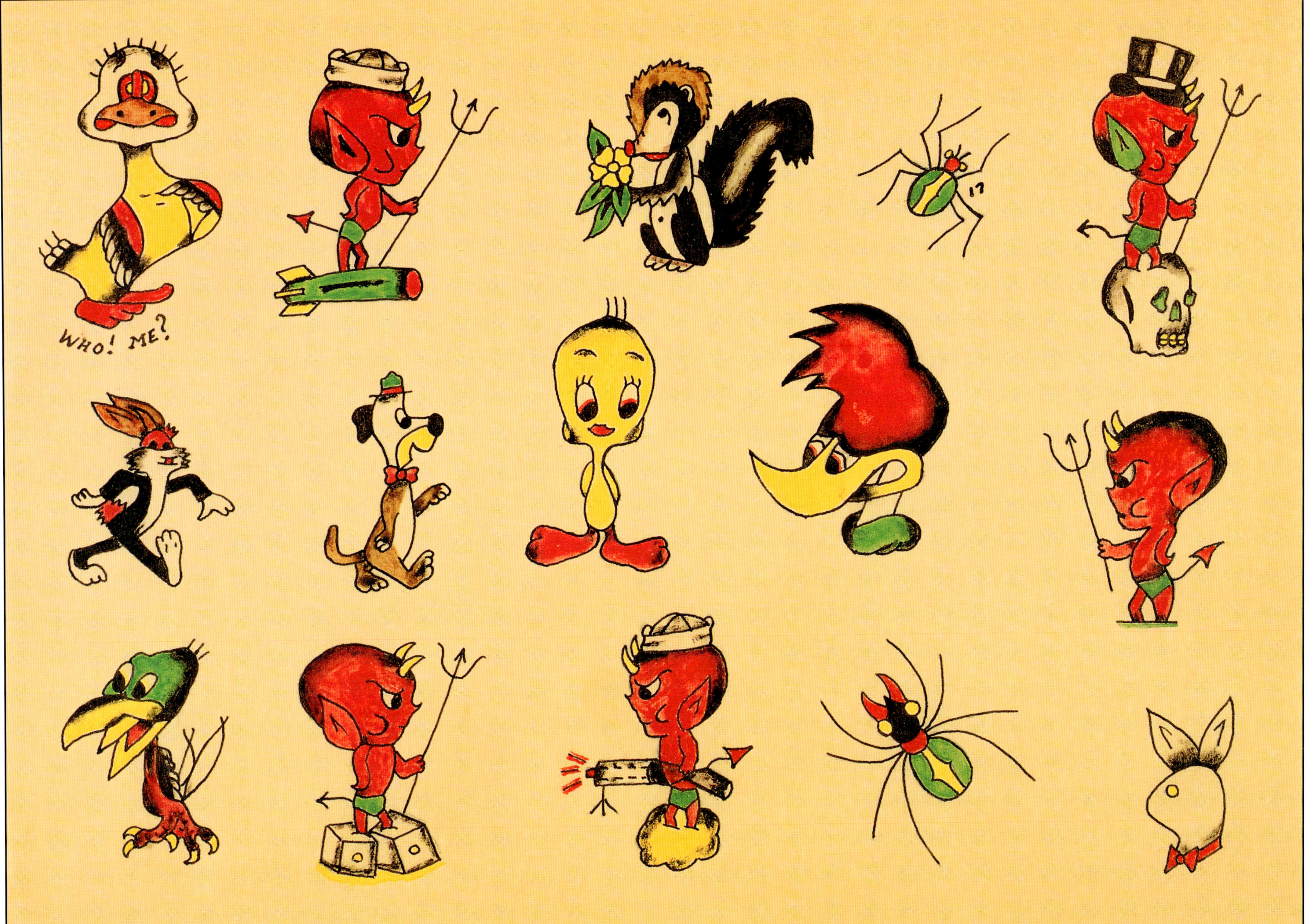
WHO! ME?
17

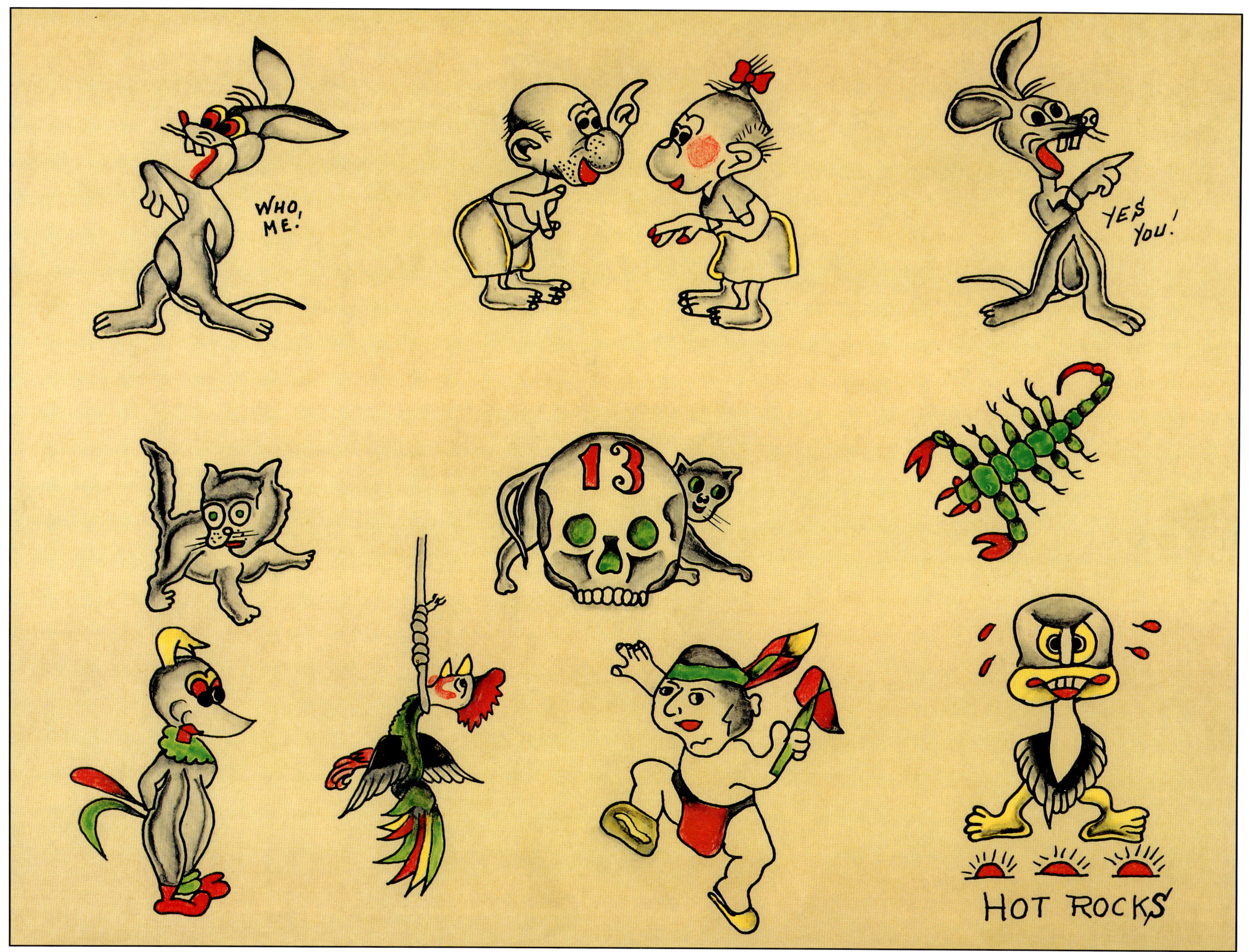
WHO, ME!
YES YOU!
13
HOT ROCKS

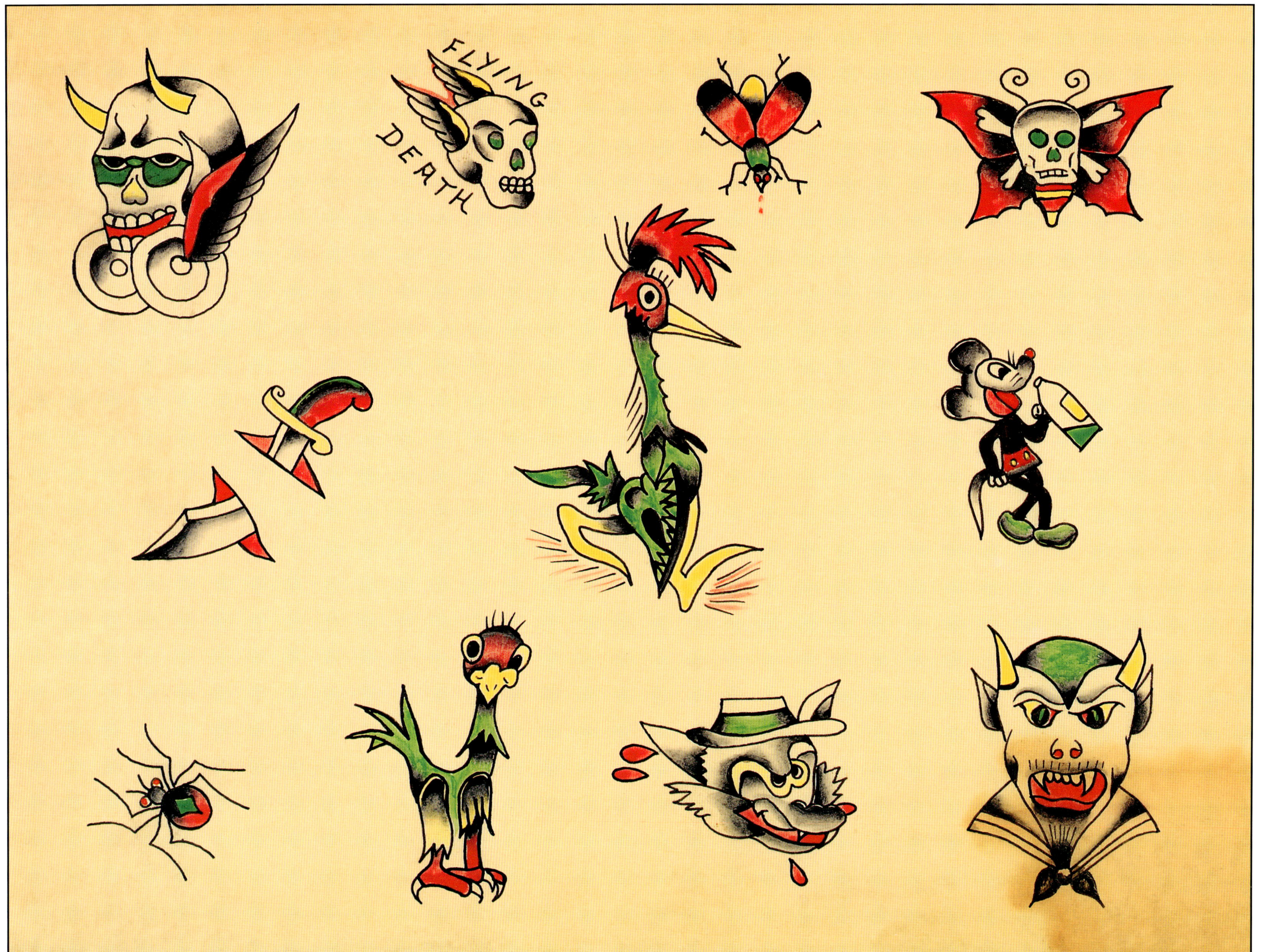
FLYING
DEATH

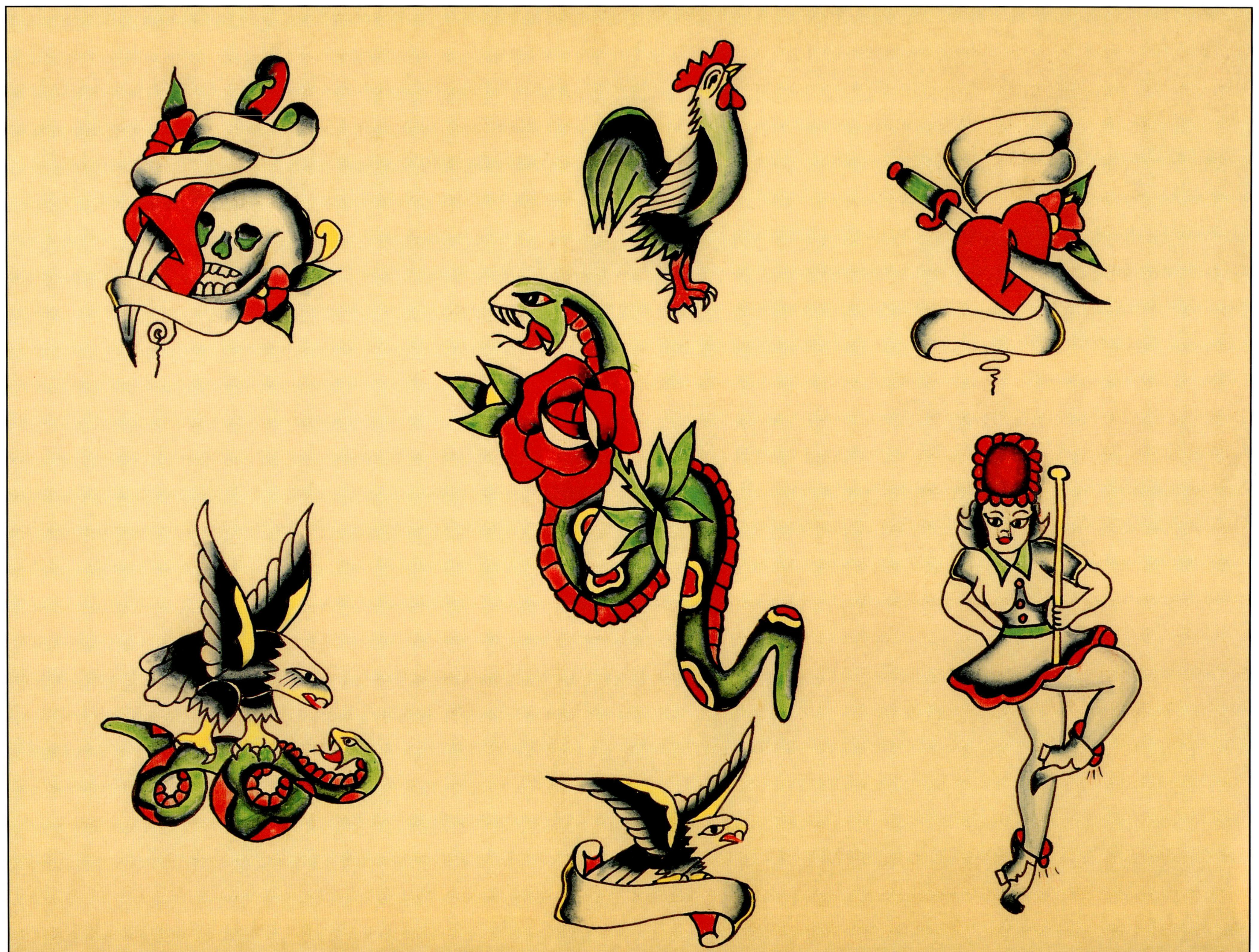

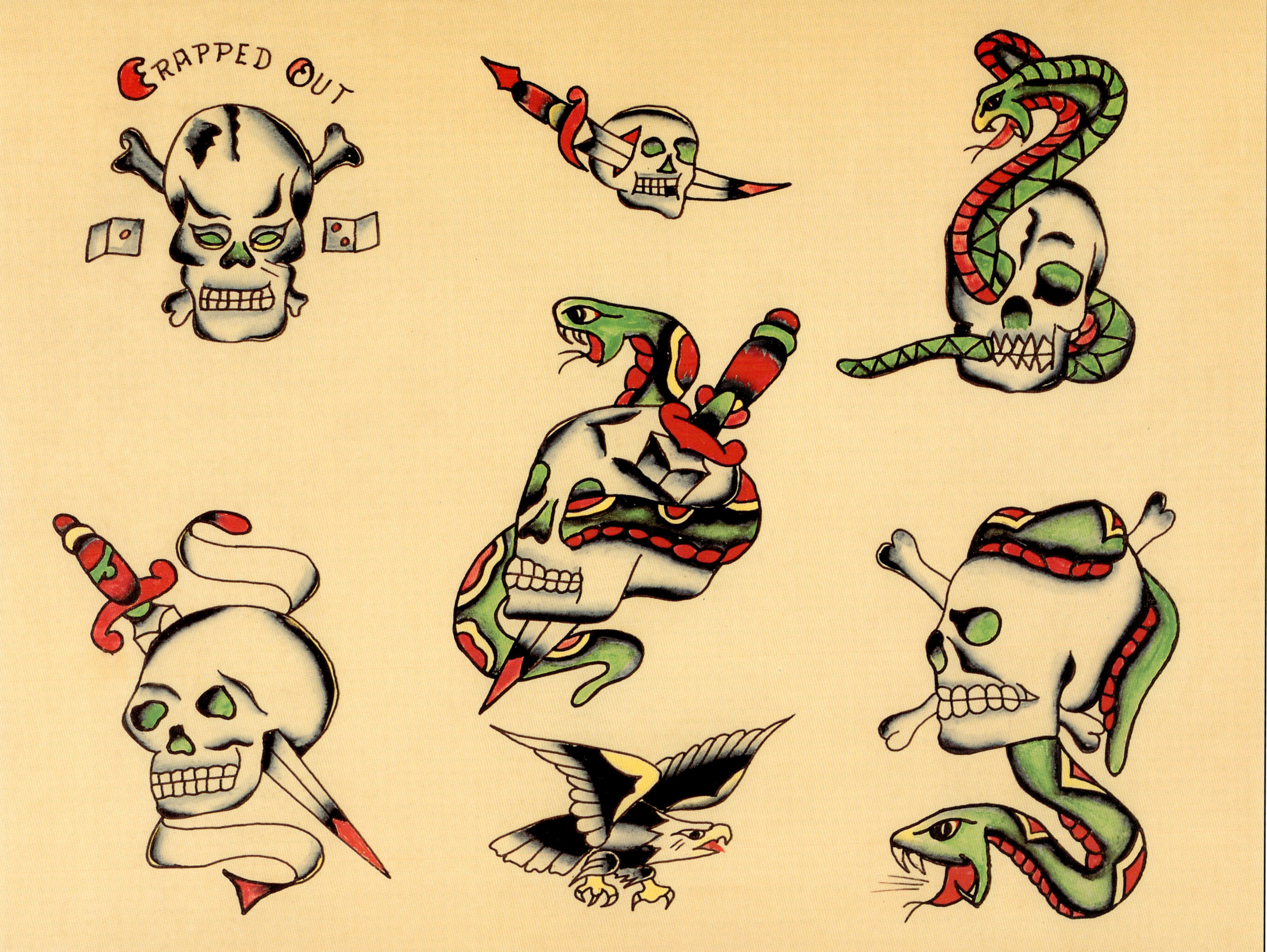
CRAPPED OUT

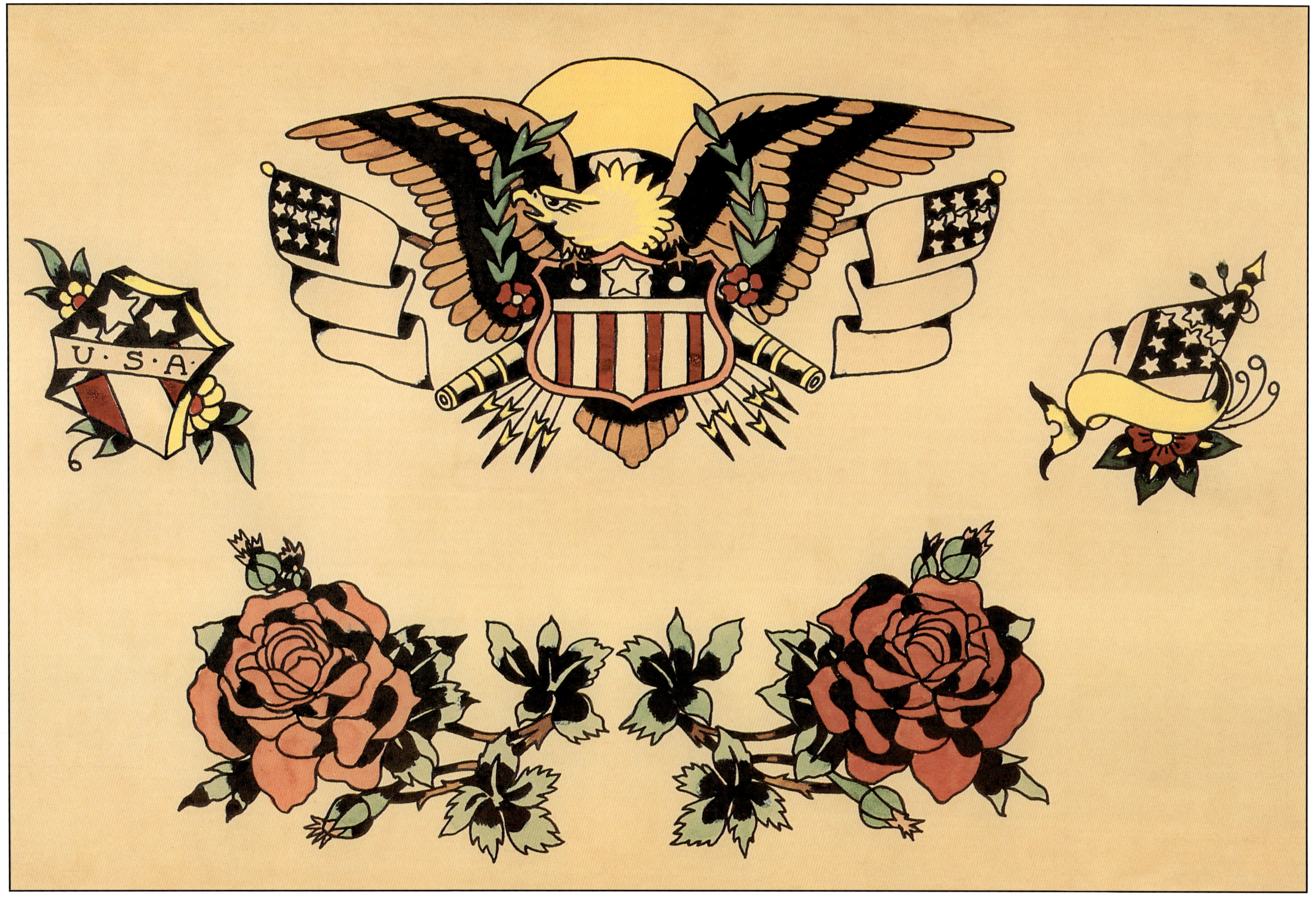
U·S·A

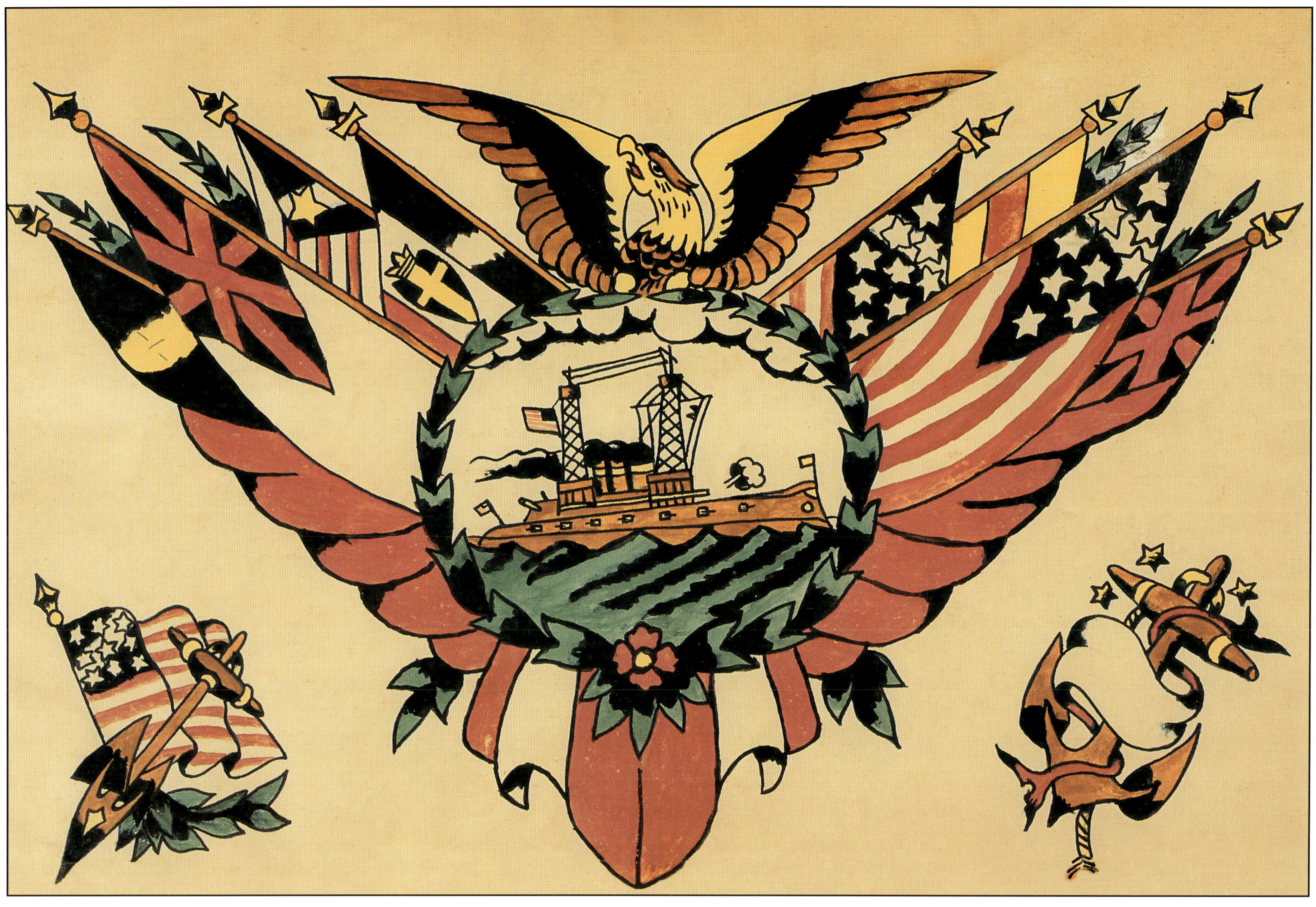

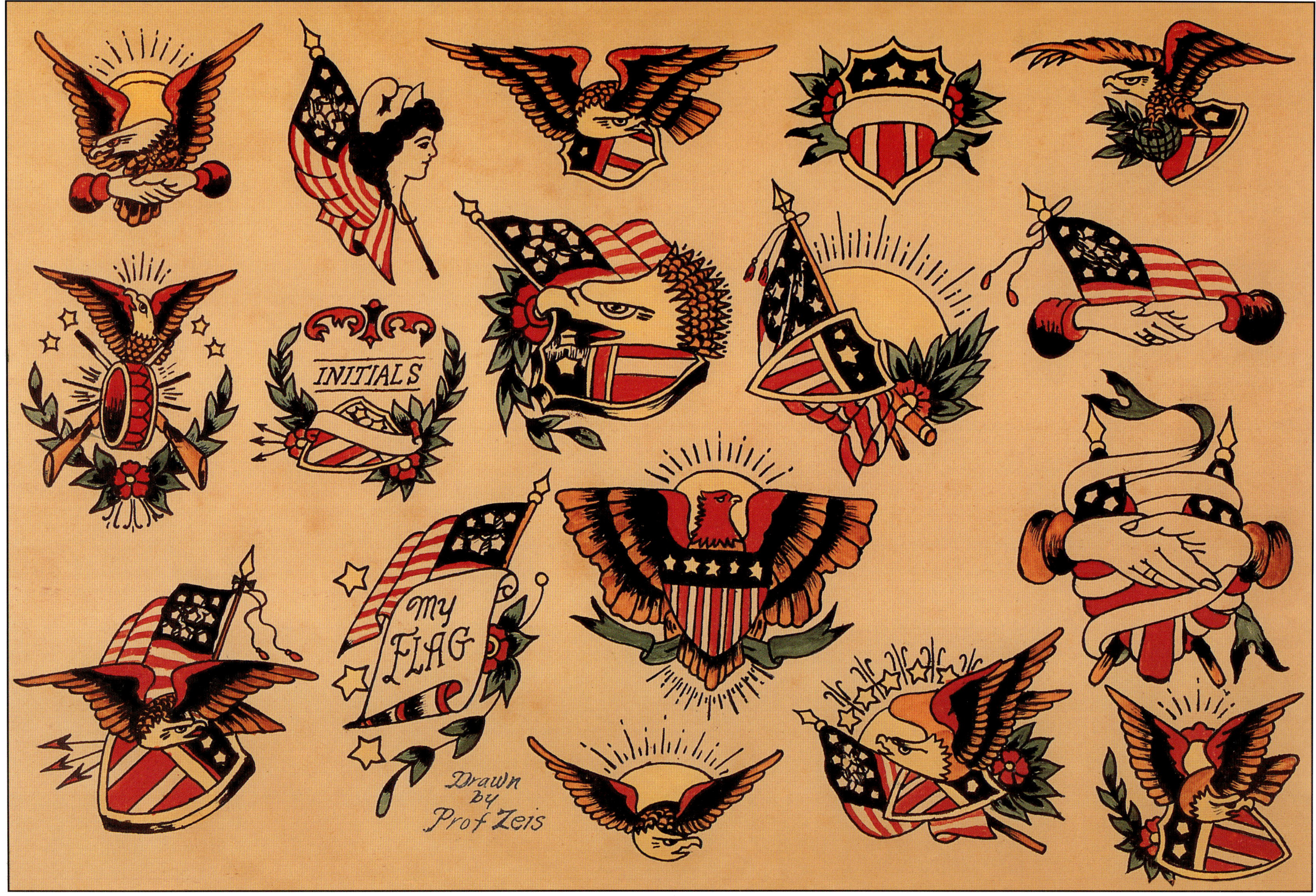
INITIALS
MY FLAG
Drawn by Prof Zeis

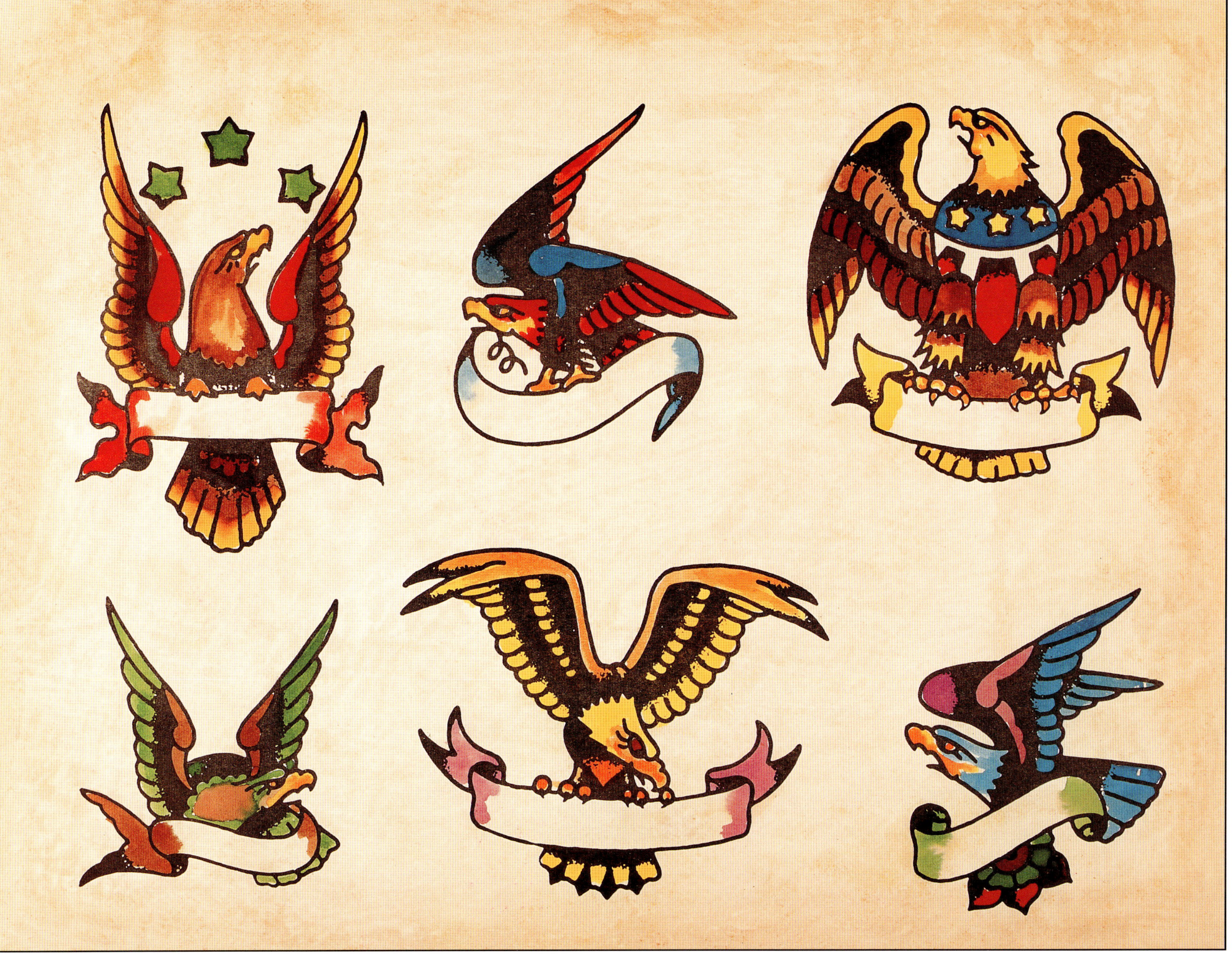

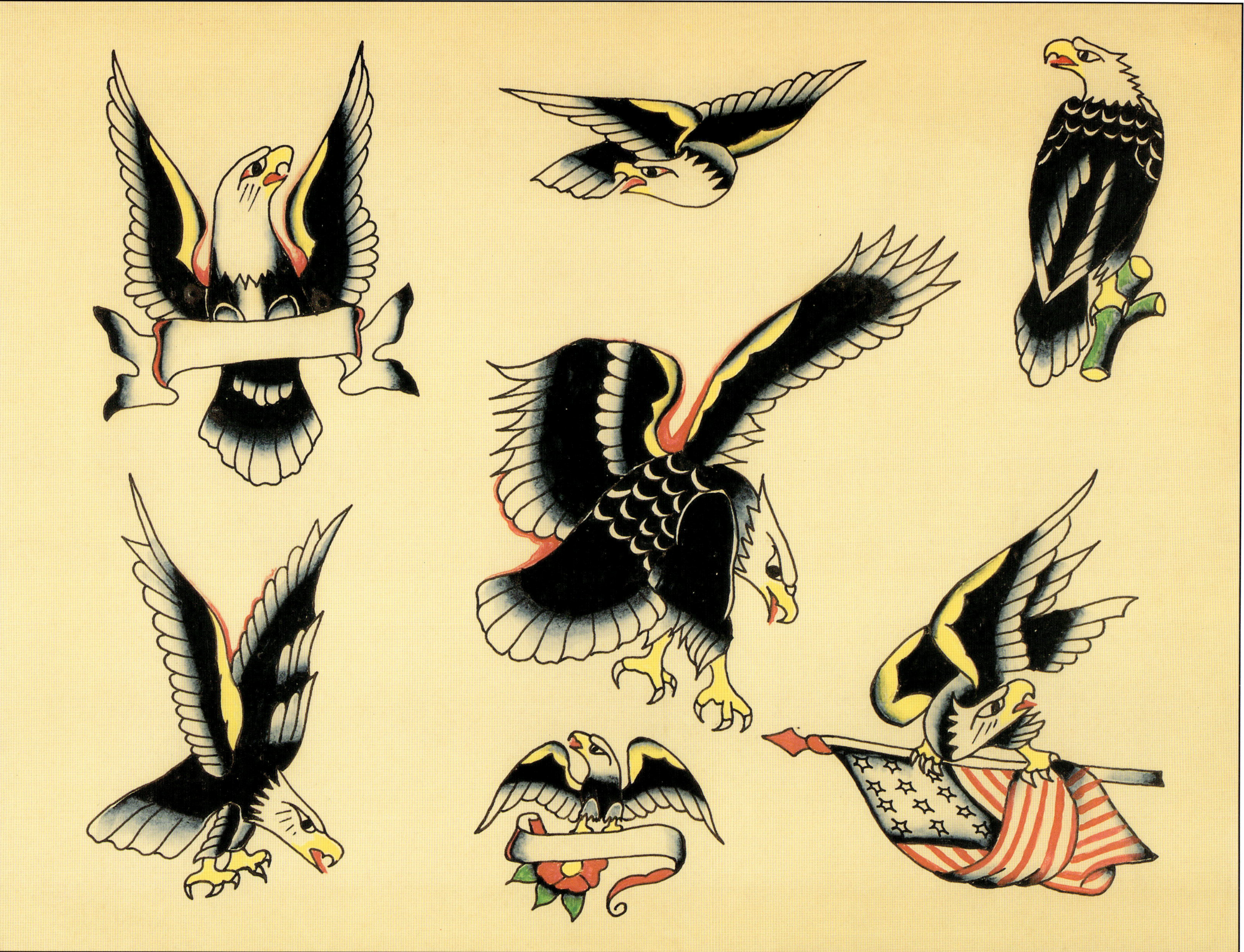

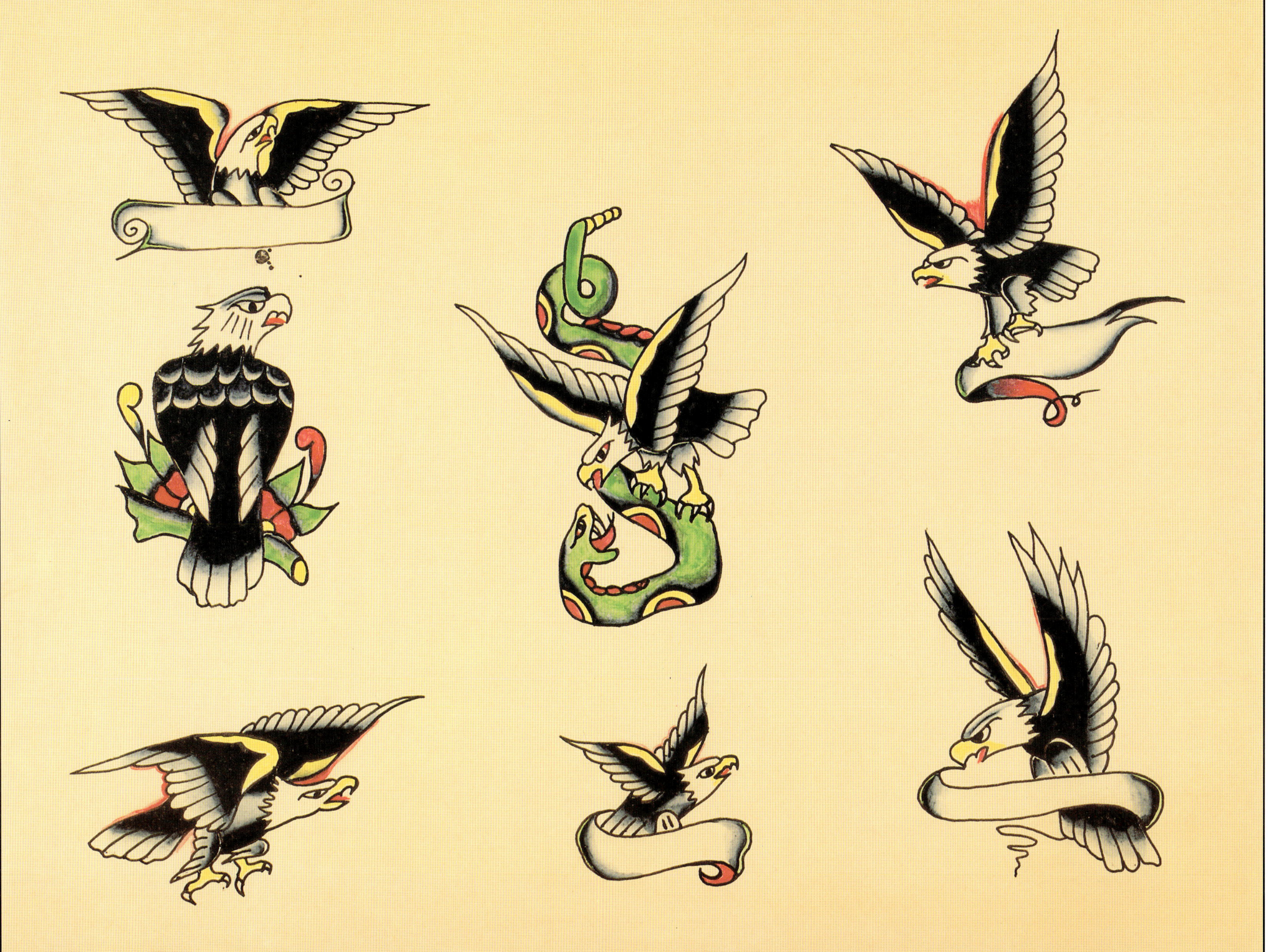

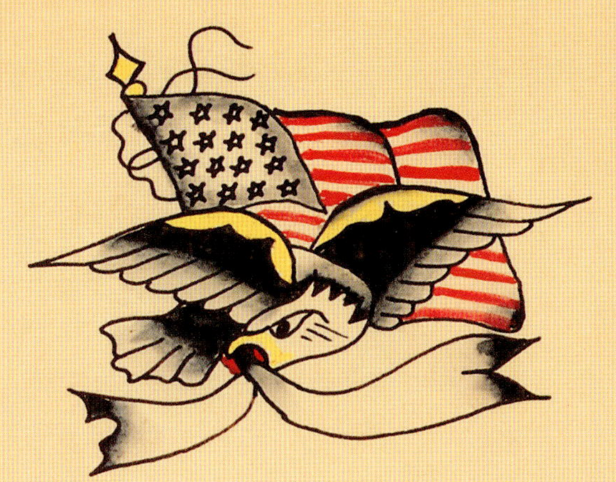
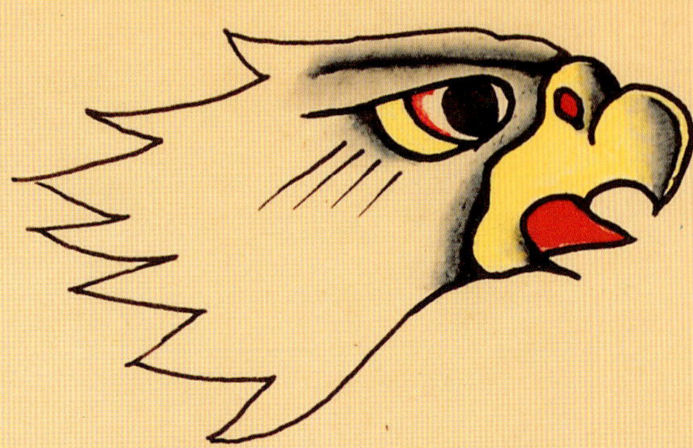
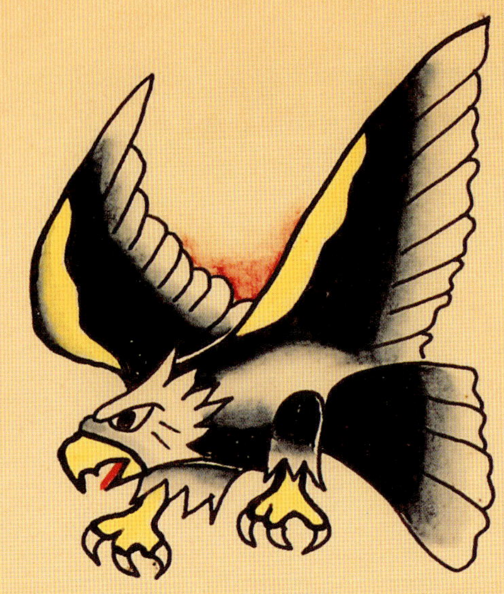
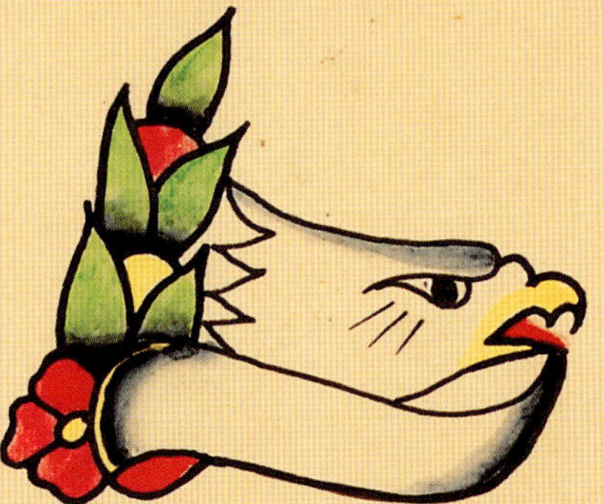
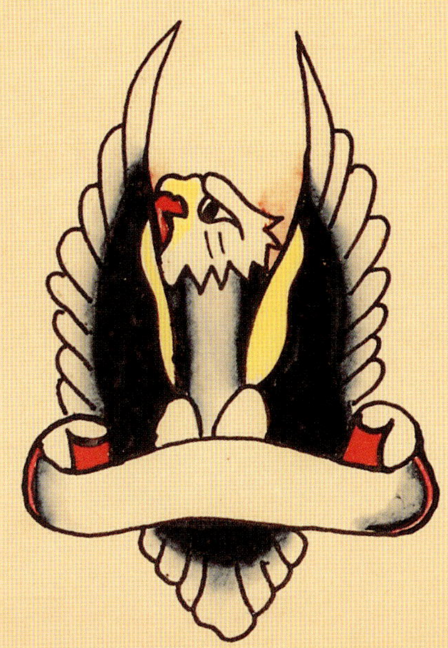
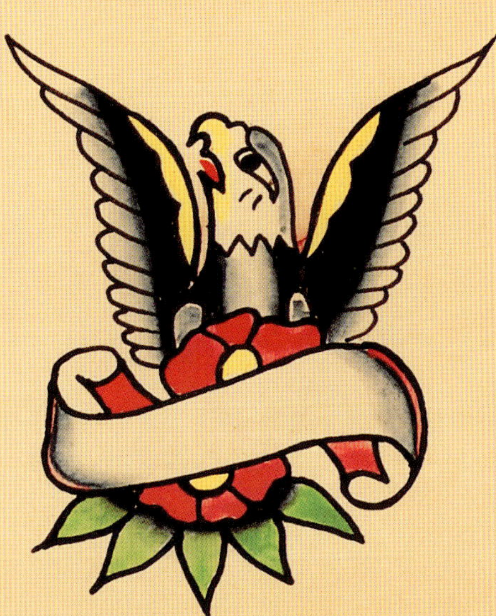
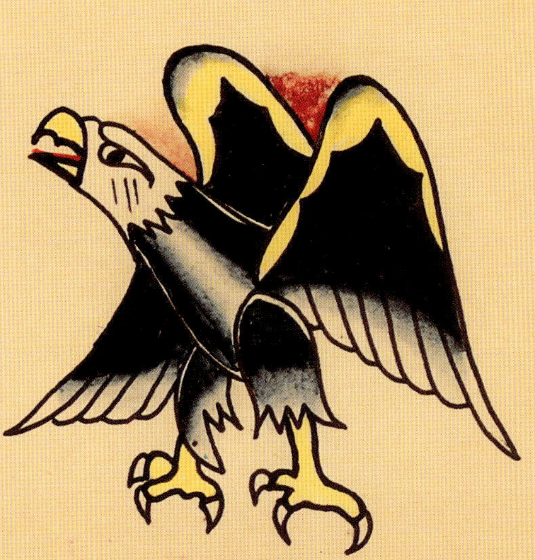

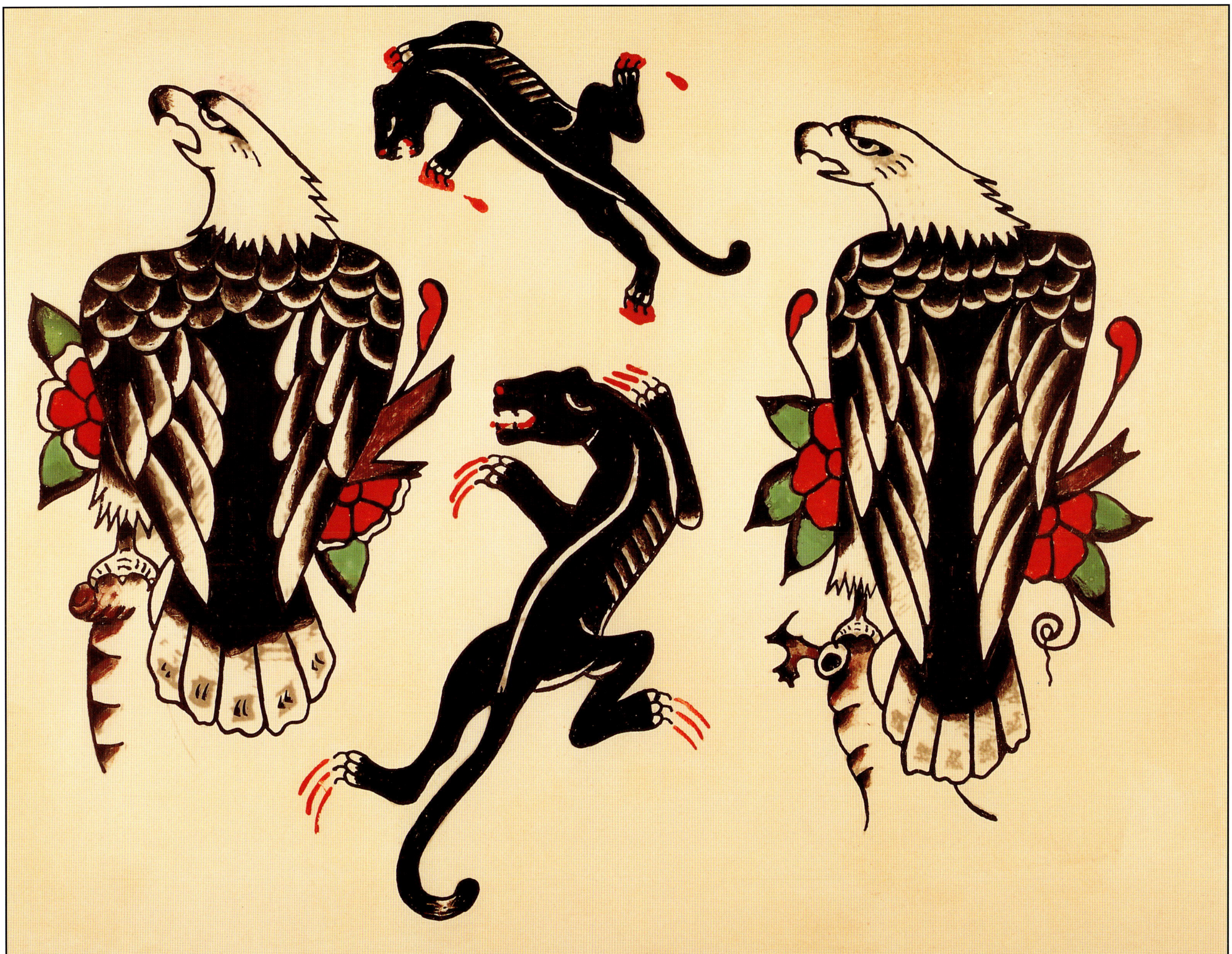

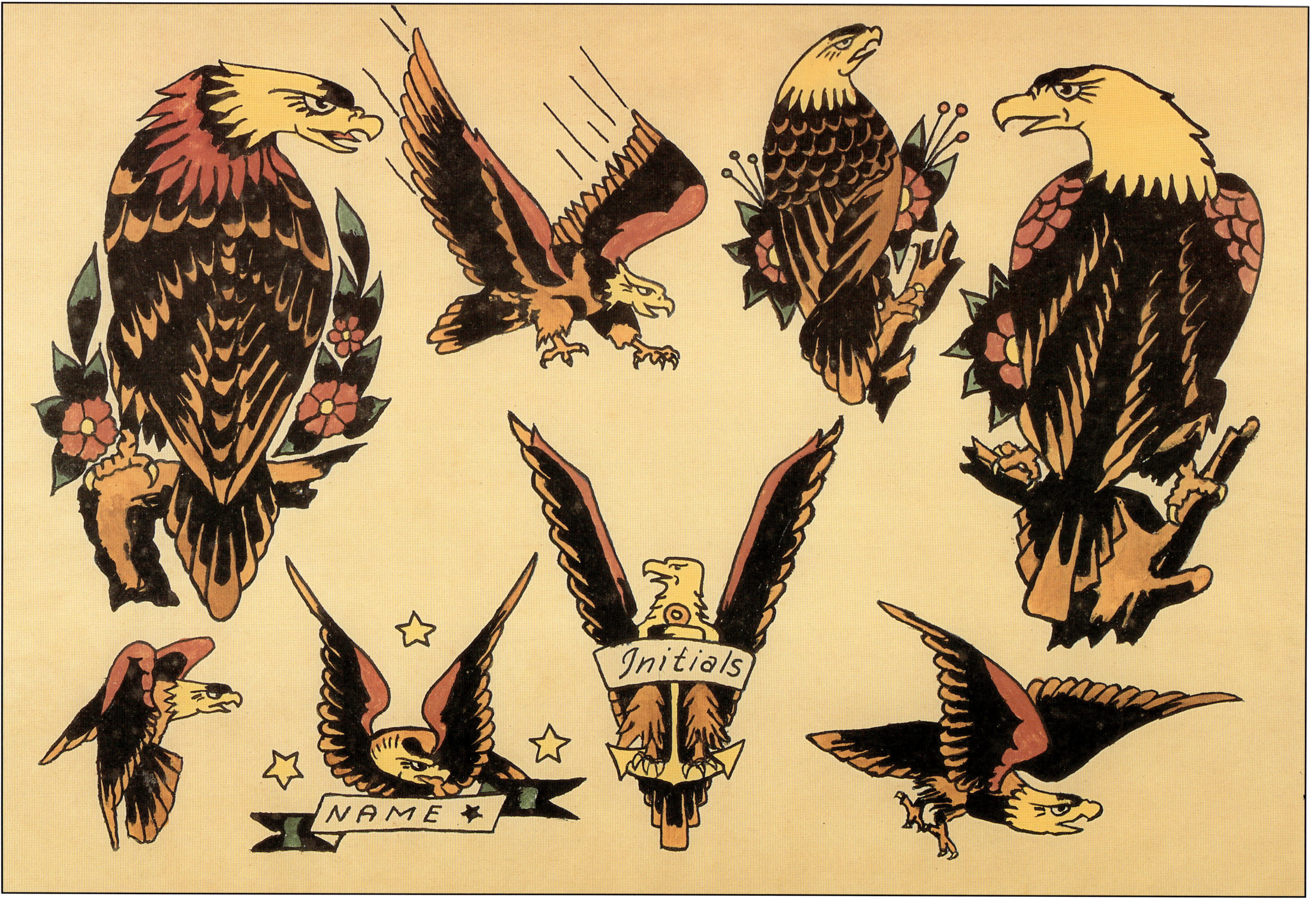
Initials
NAME ★

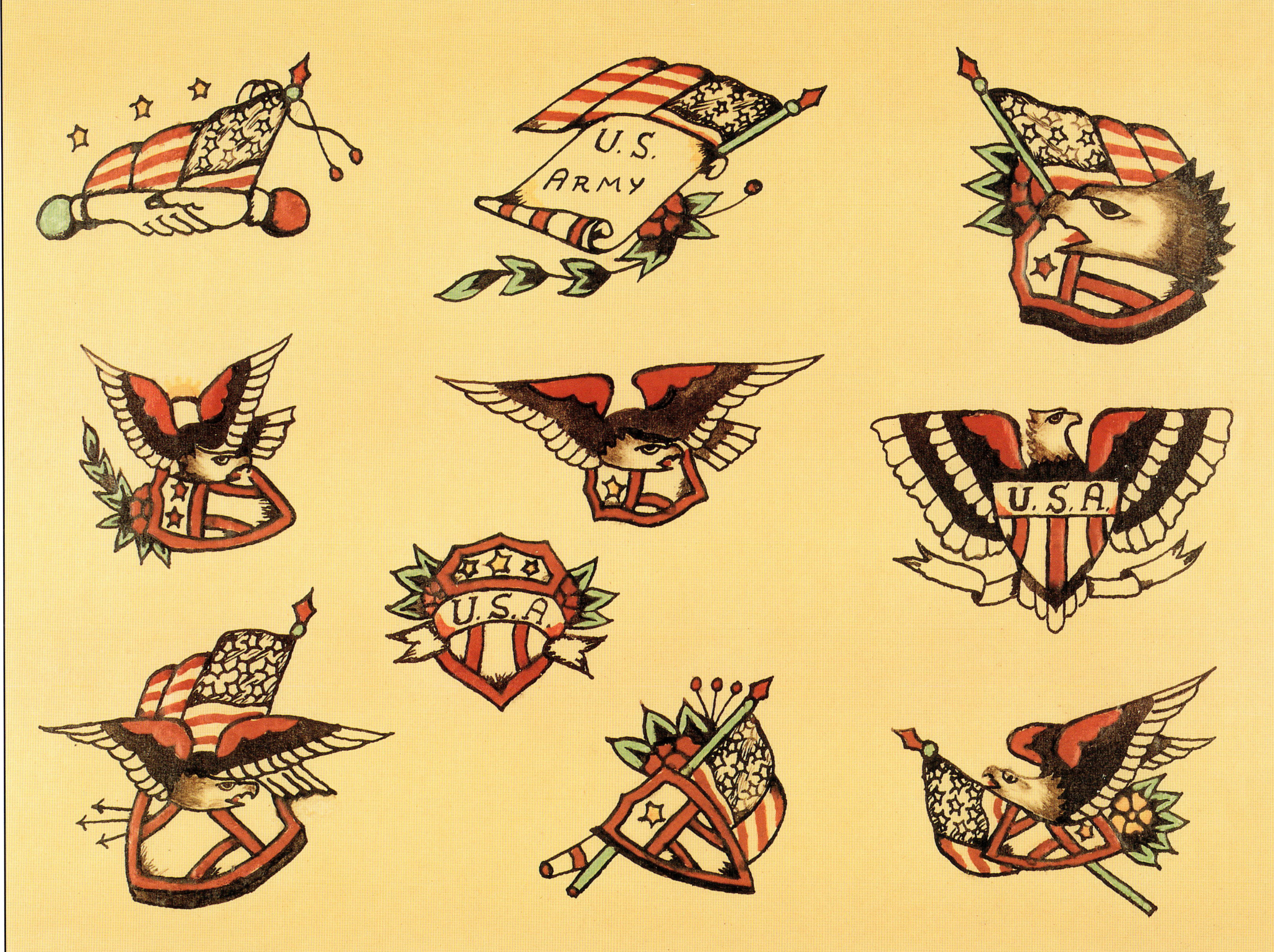
U.S.
ARMY
U.S.A.
U.S.A

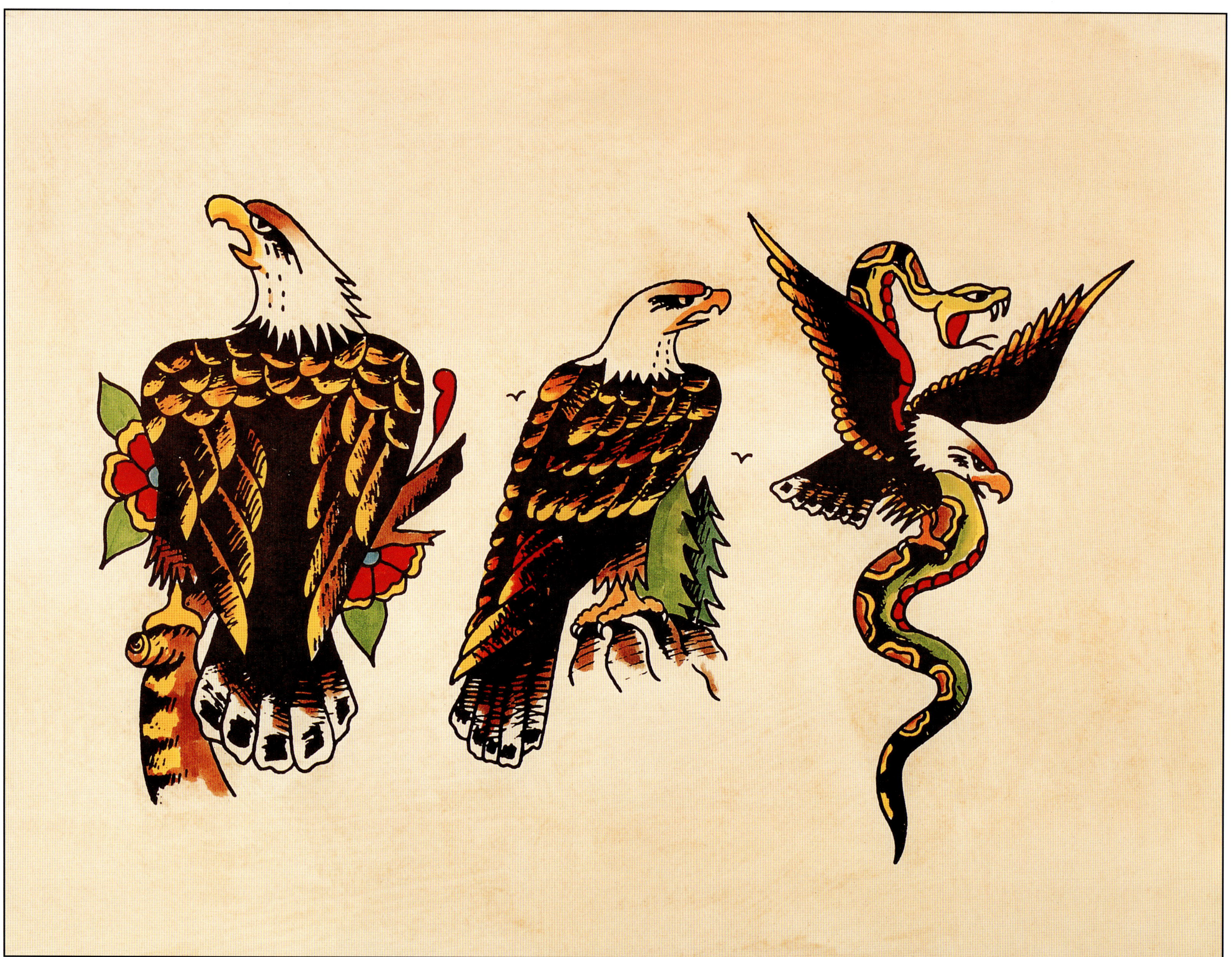

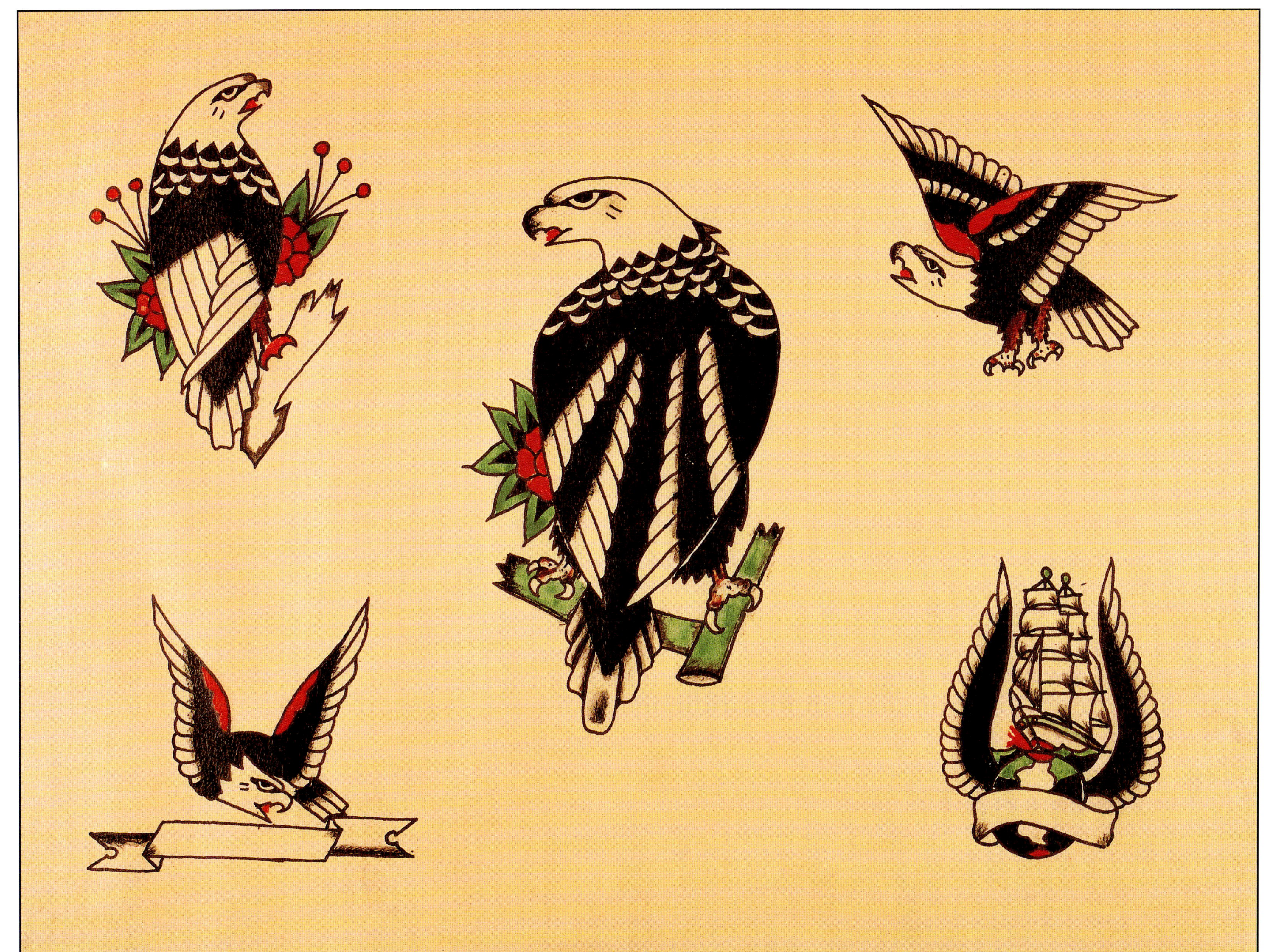

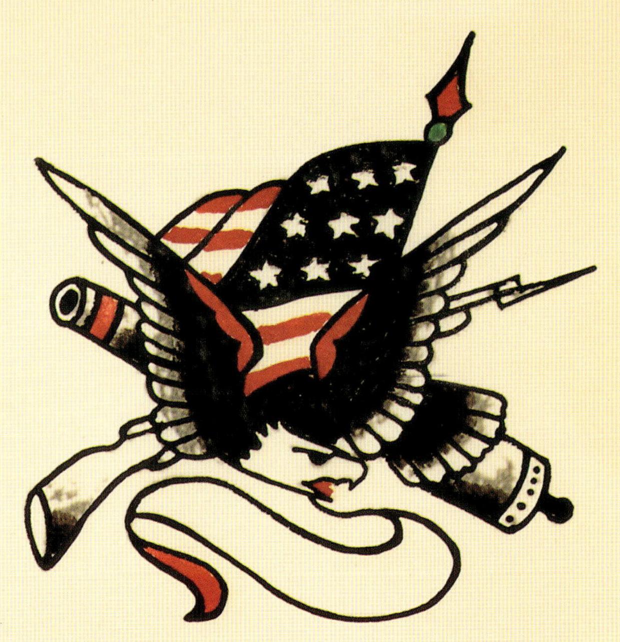
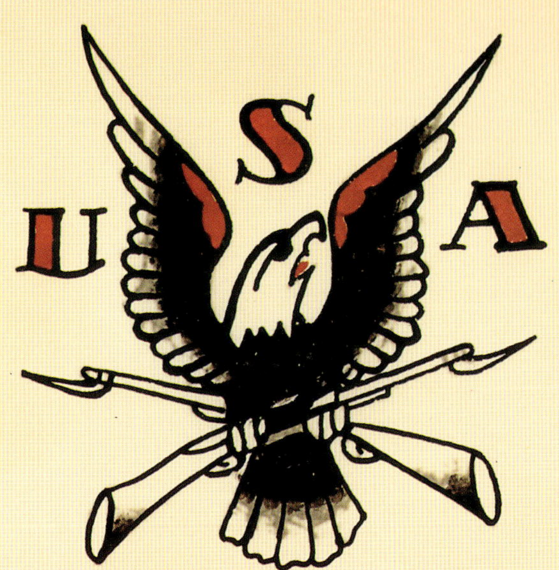
U S A
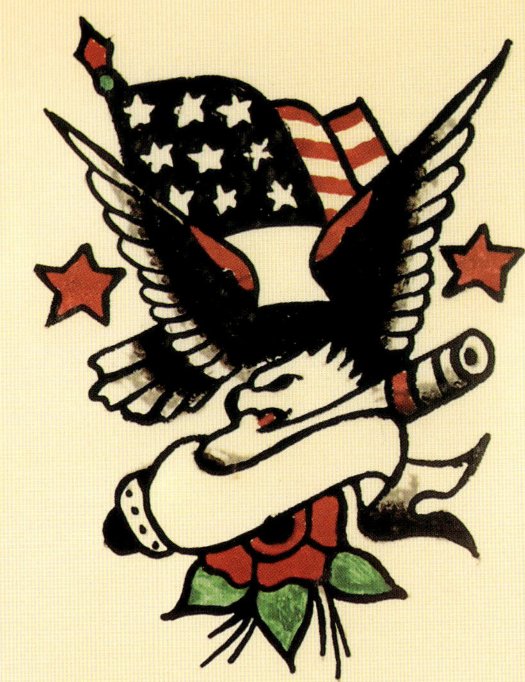
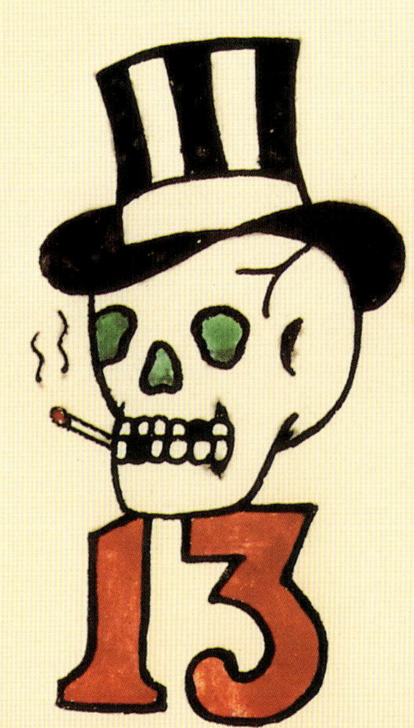
13
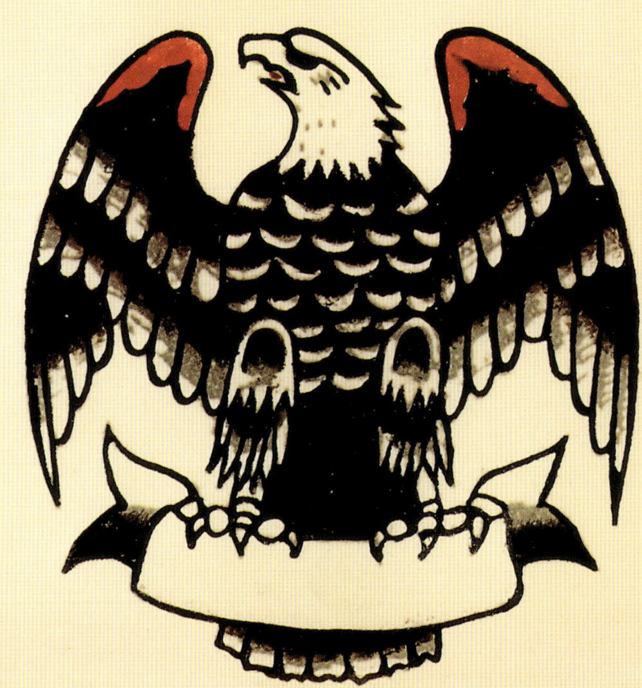
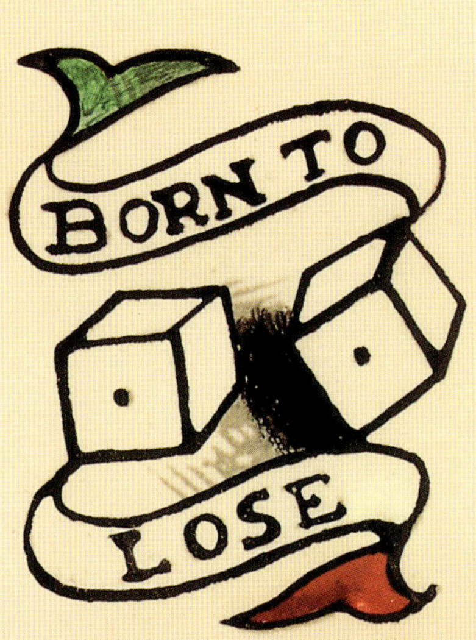
BORN TO
LOSE

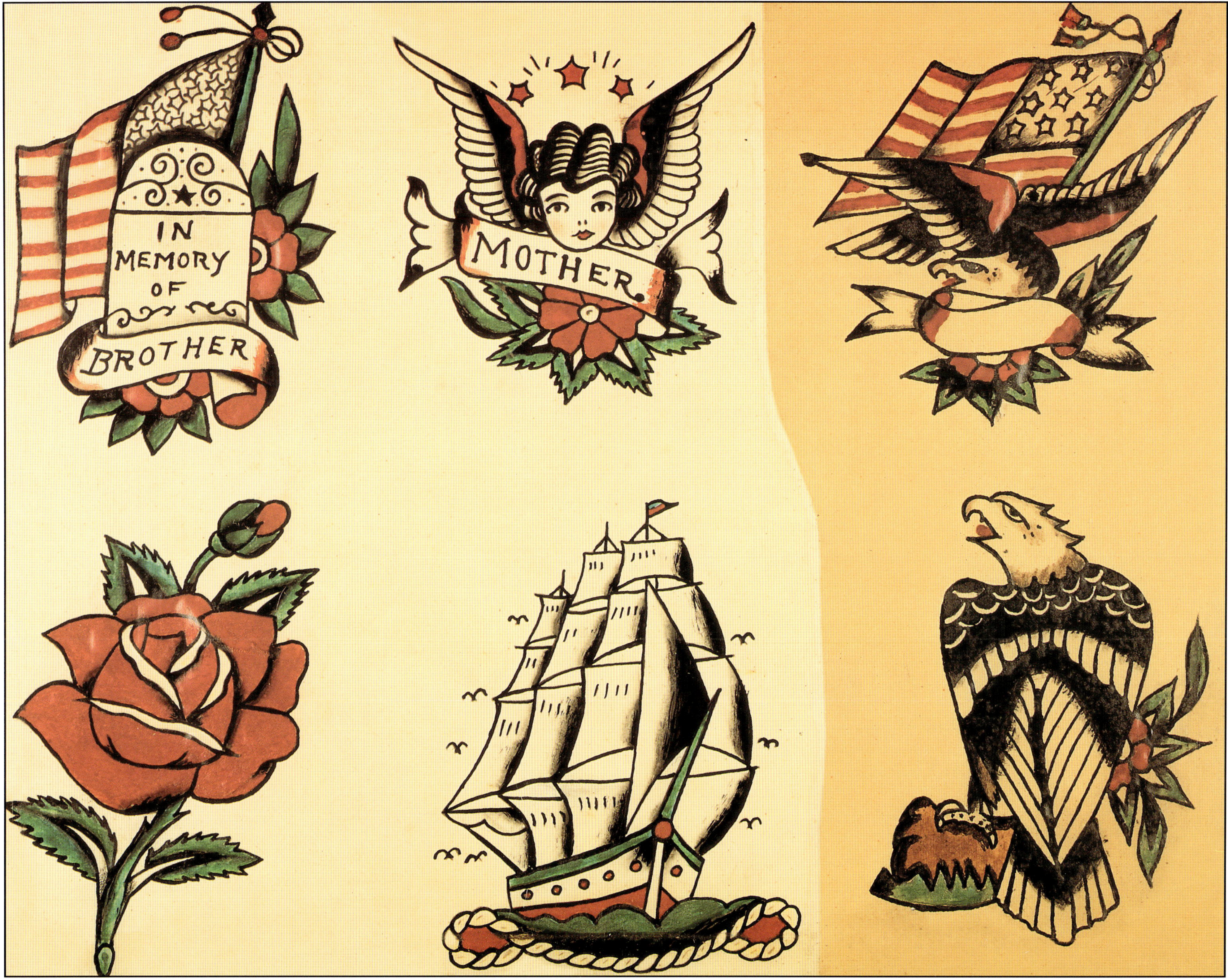
IN MEMORY OF
BROTHER
MOTHER

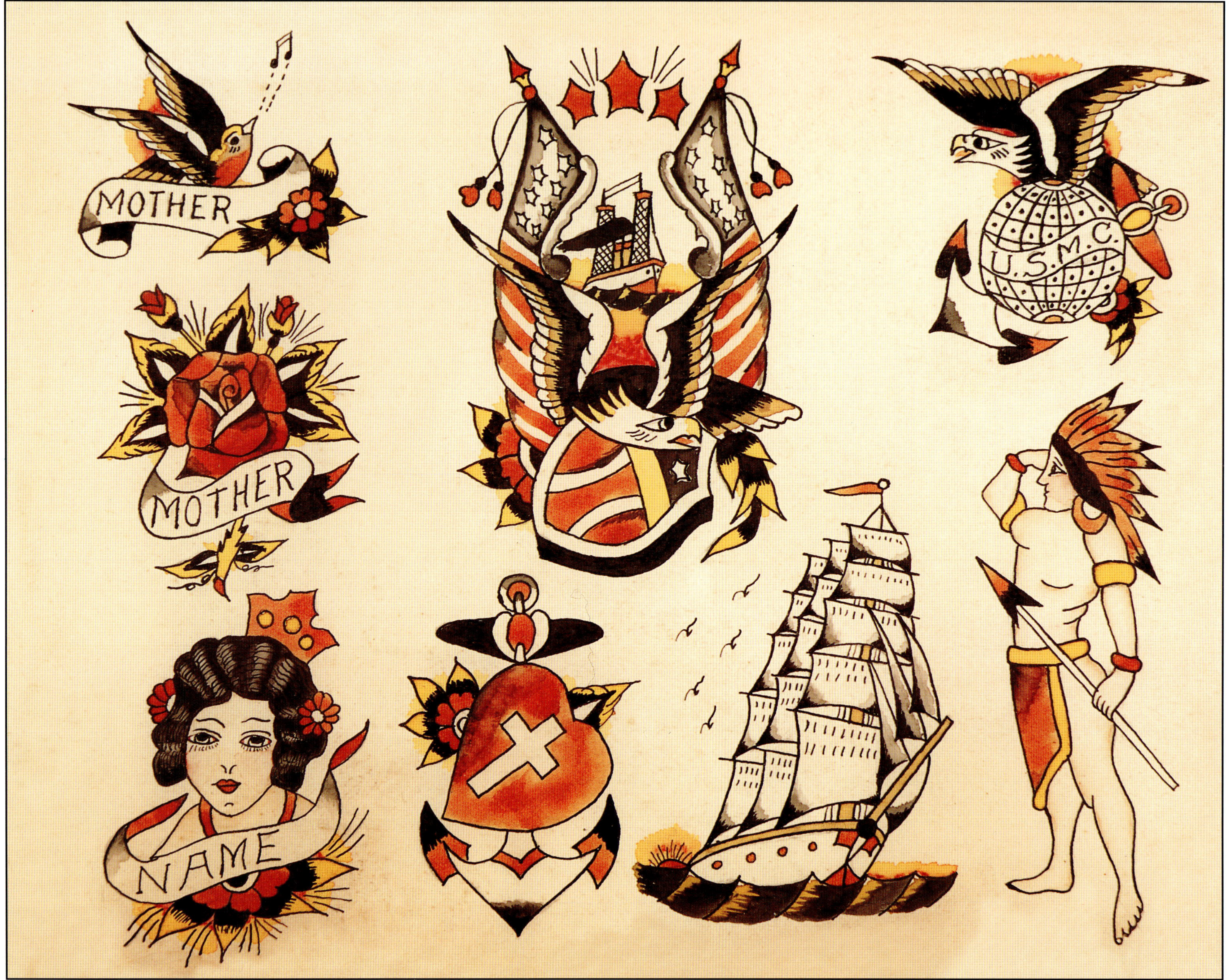
MOTHER
MOTHER
U.S.M.C.
NAME

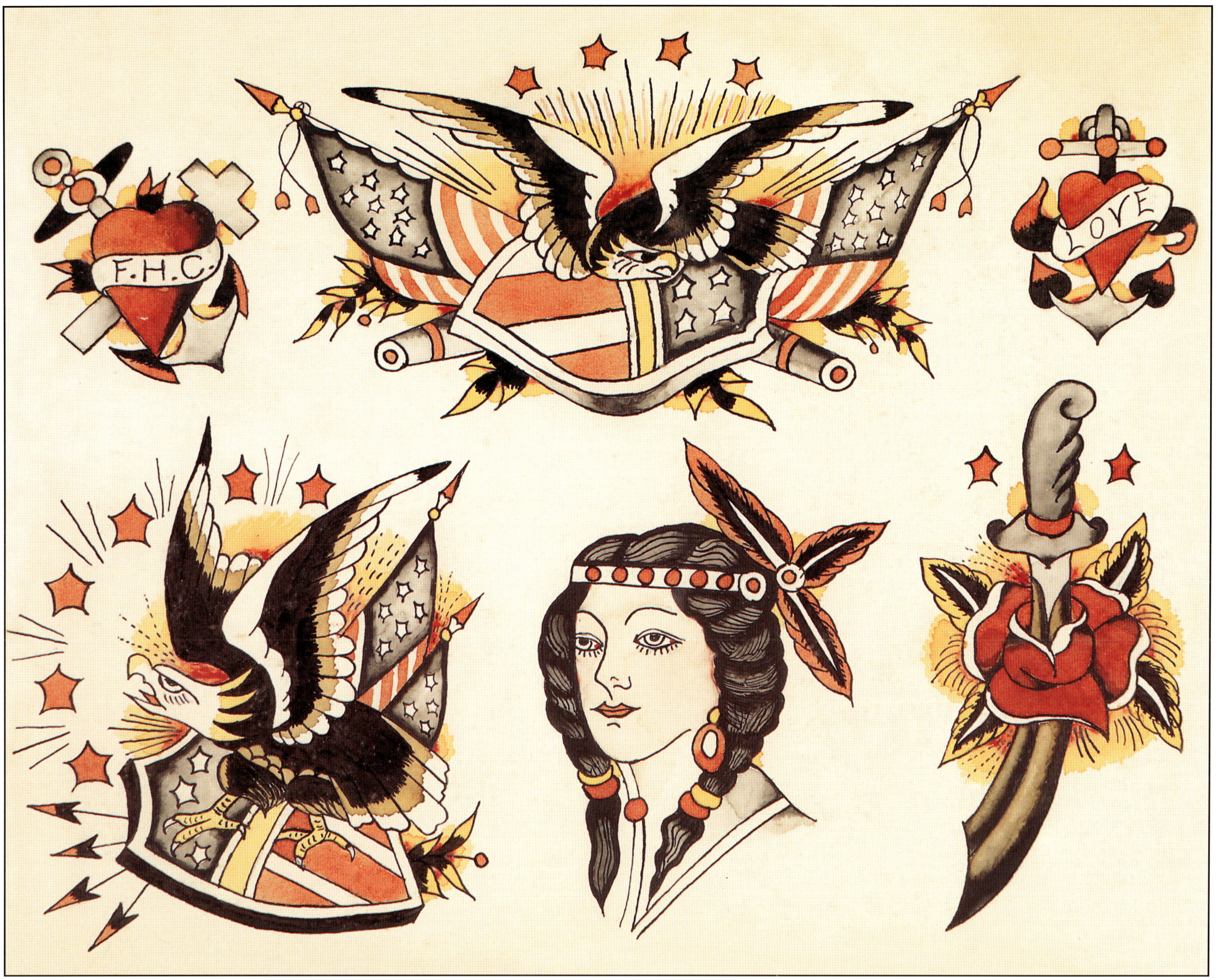
F.H.C.
LOVE

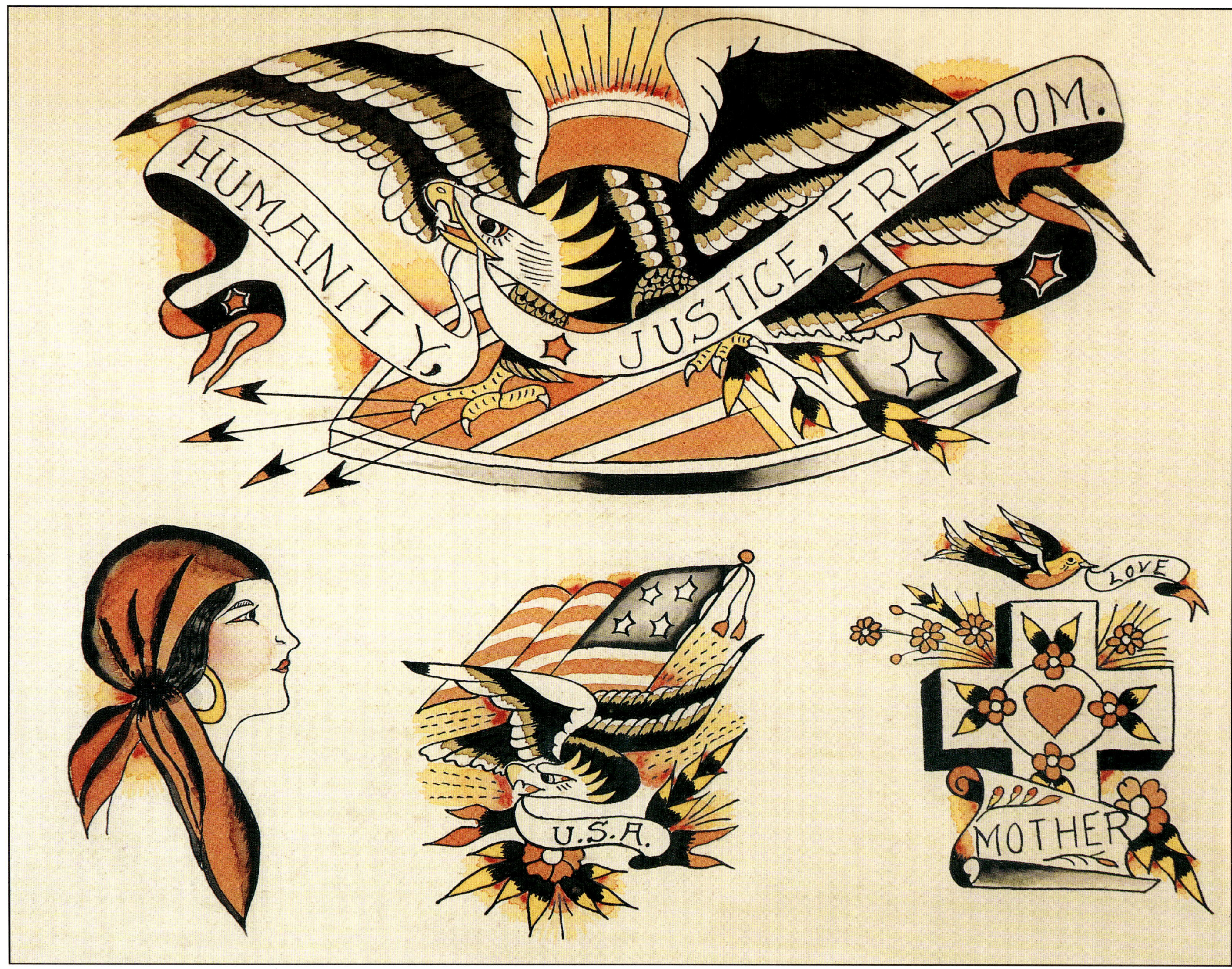
HUMANITY
JUSTICE, FREEDOM.
U.S.A.
LOVE
MOTHER

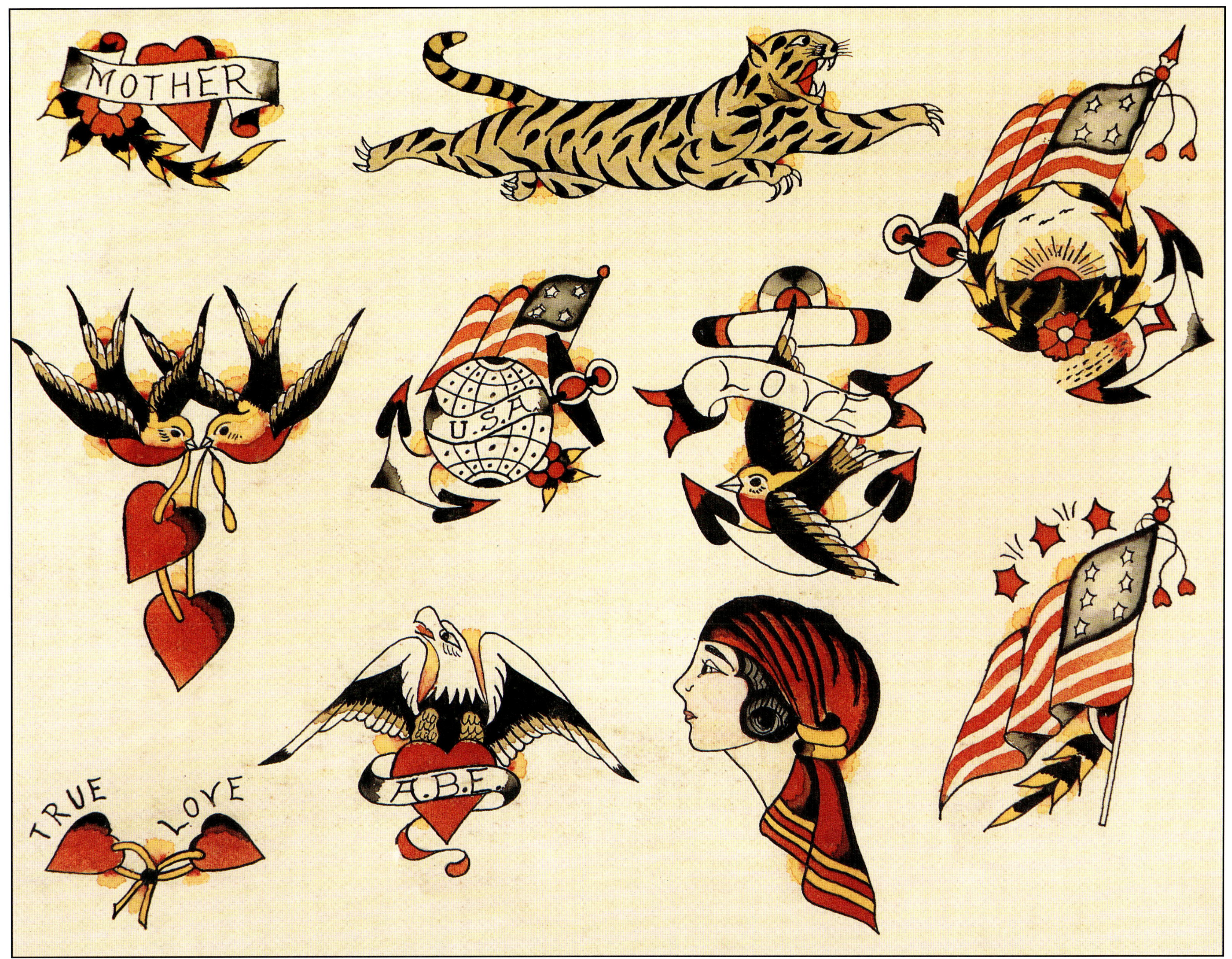
MOTHER
U.S.A.
LOVE
TRUE LOVE
A.B.E.

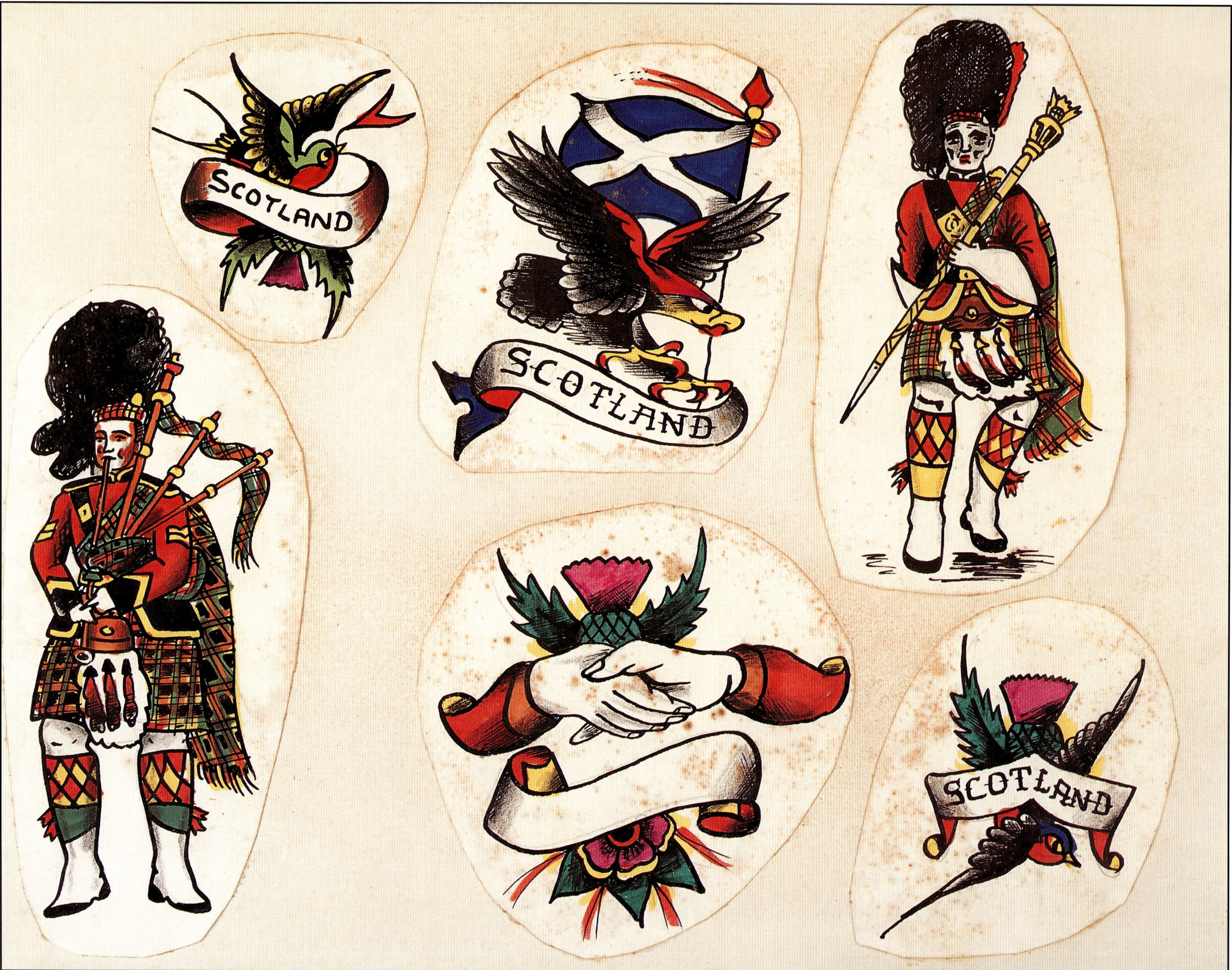
SCOTLAND
SCOTLAND
SCOTLAND

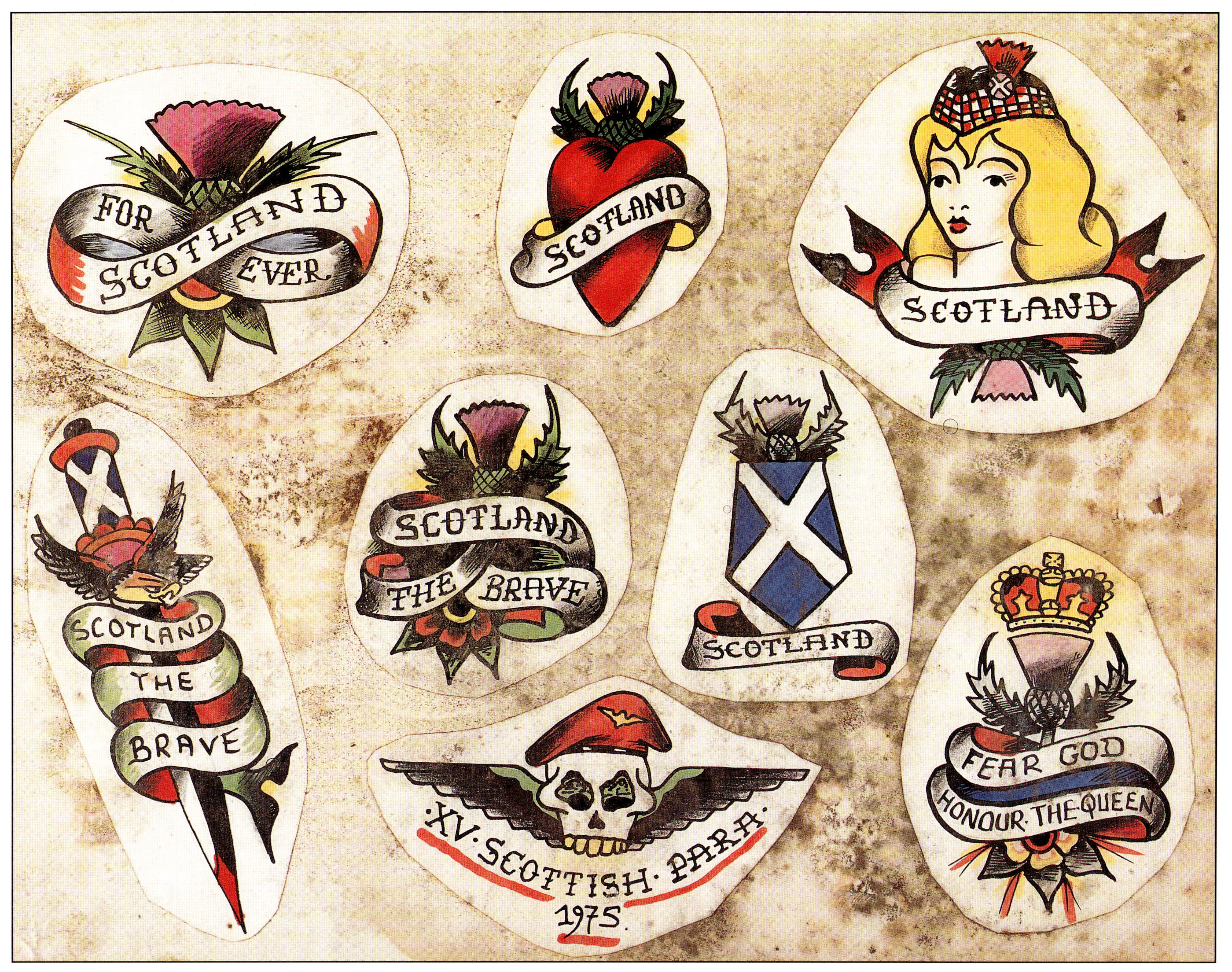

FOR SCOTLAND EVER
SCOTLAND
SCOTLAND
SCOTLAND THE BRAVE
SCOTLAND THE BRAVE
SCOTLAND
FEAR GOD
HONOUR THE QUEEN
·XV·SCOTTISH·PARA·
1975.

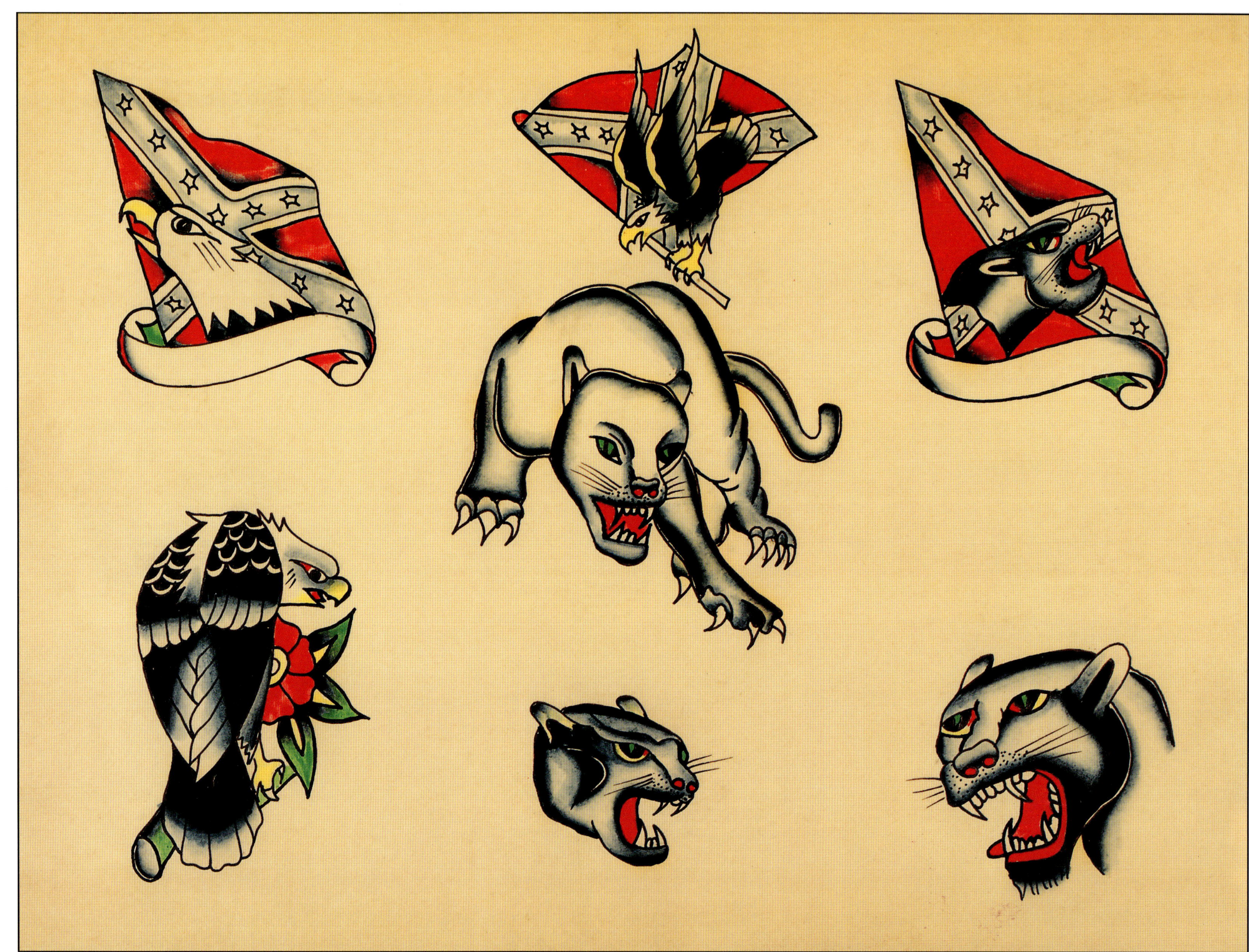

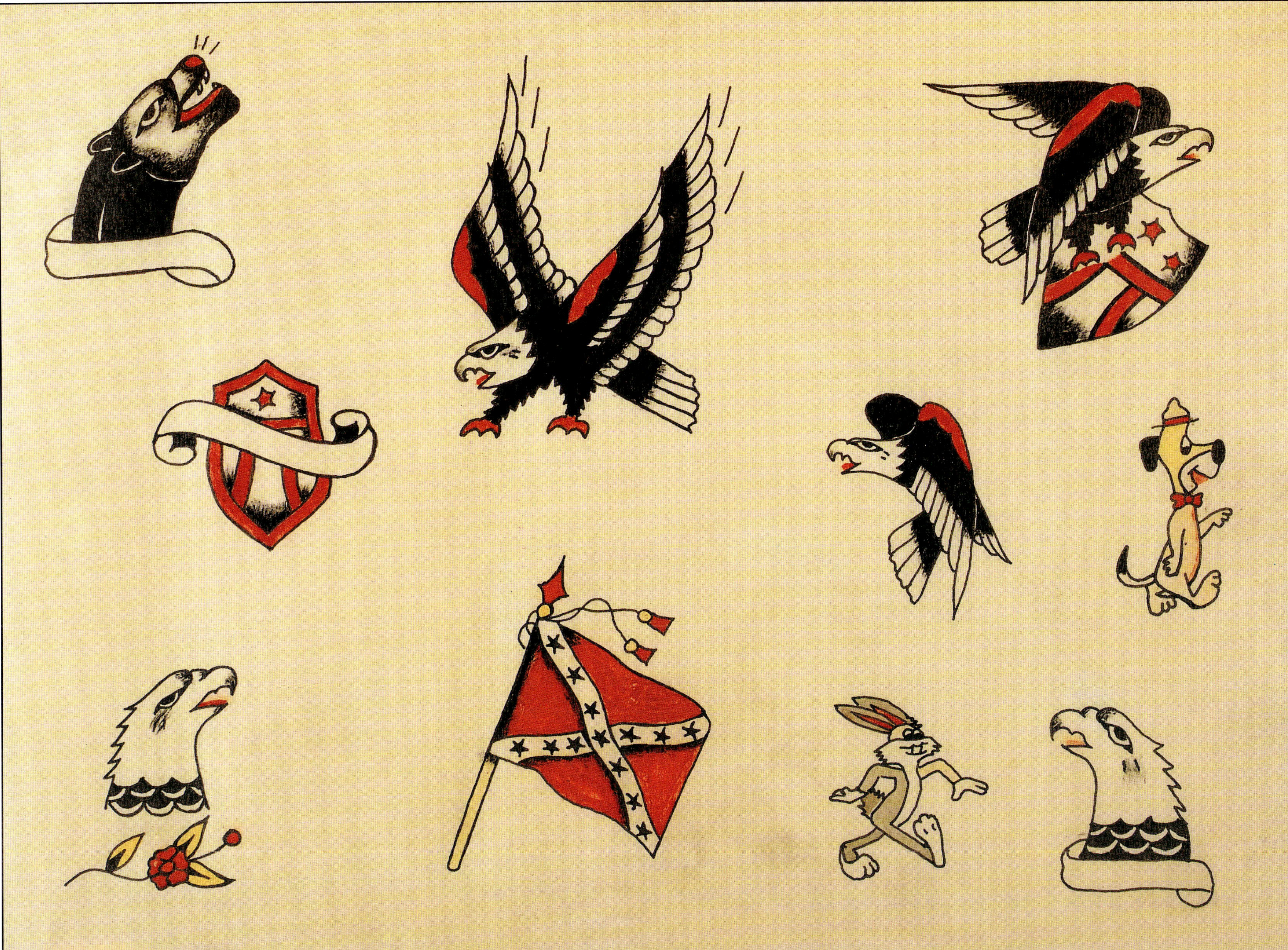

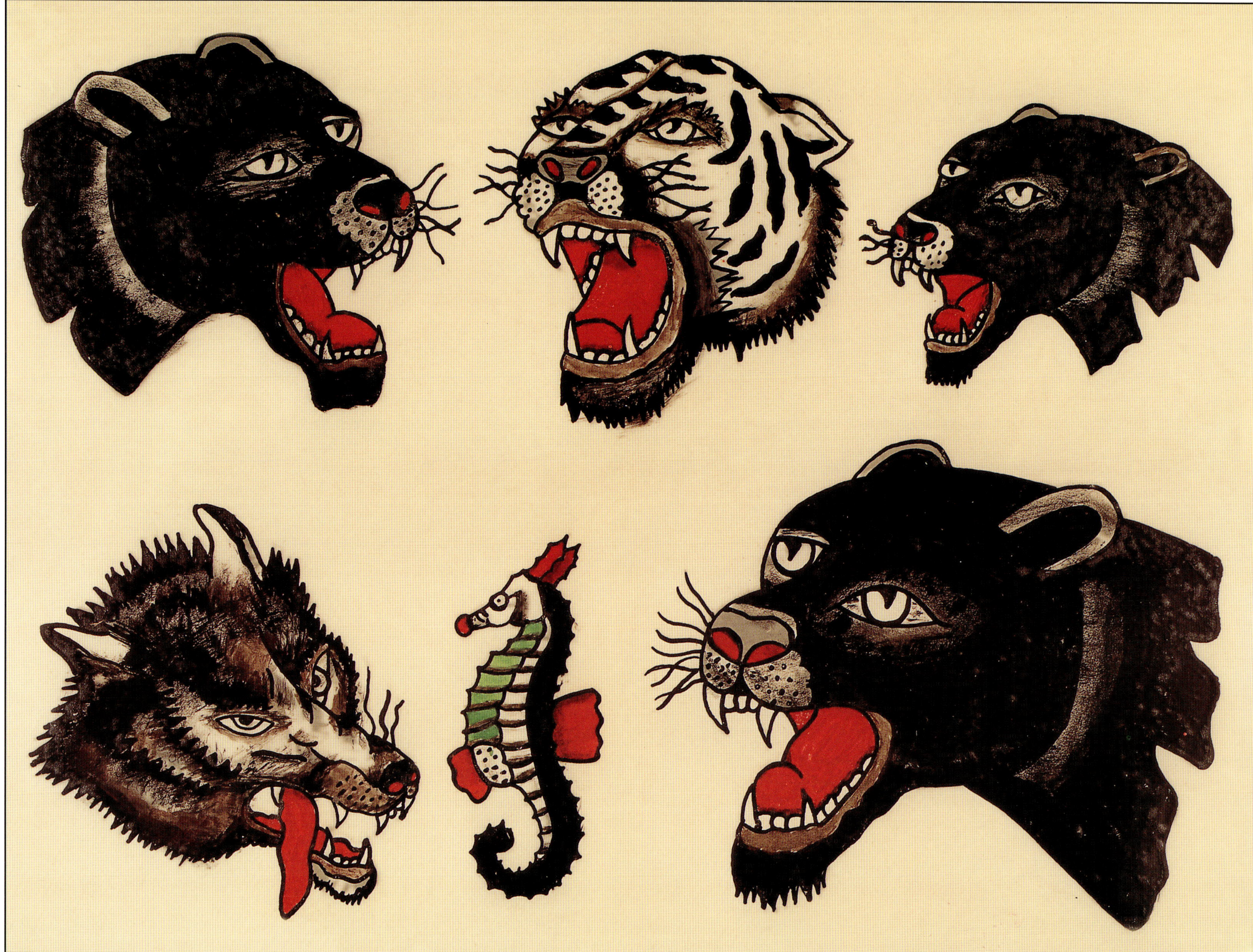

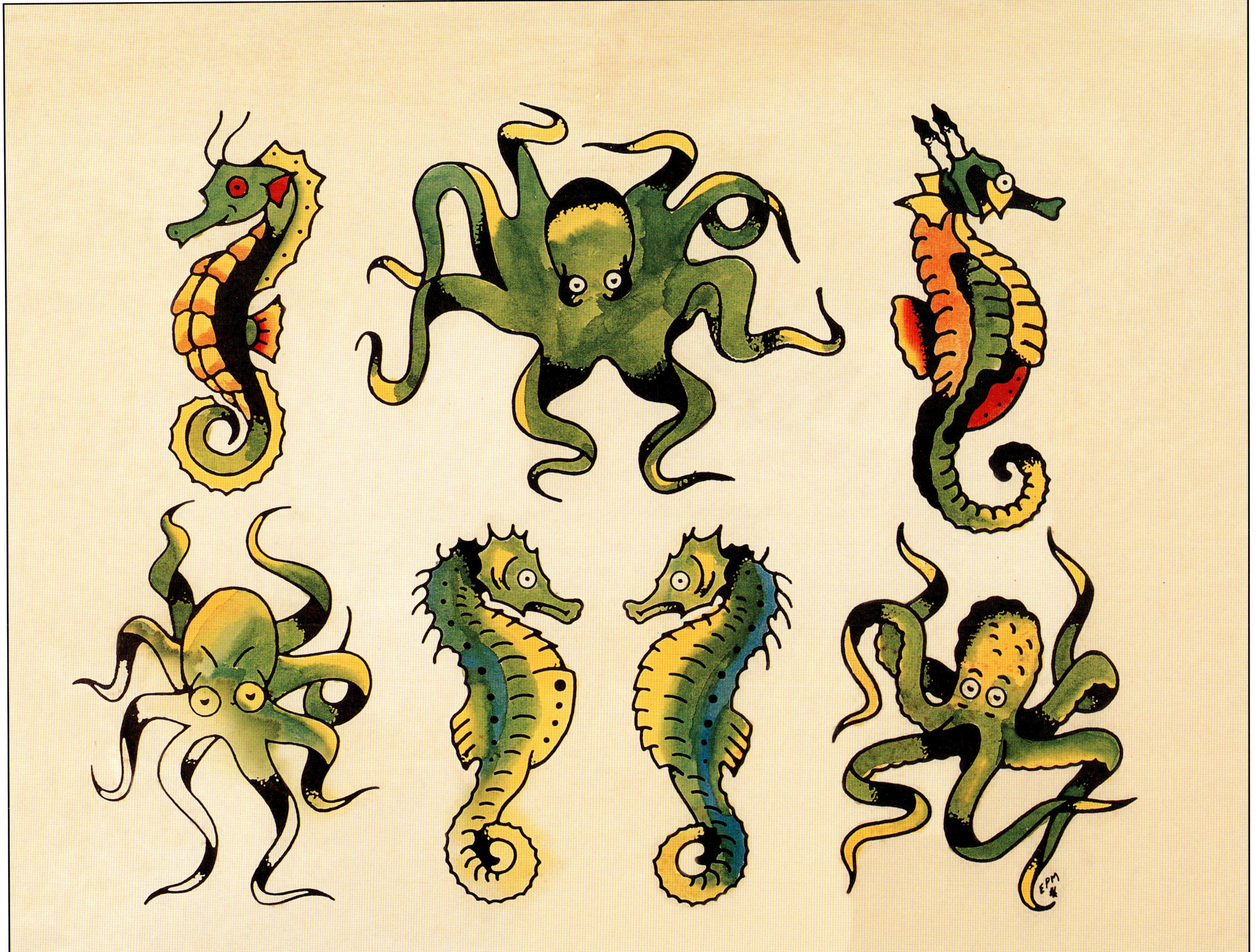
EPM

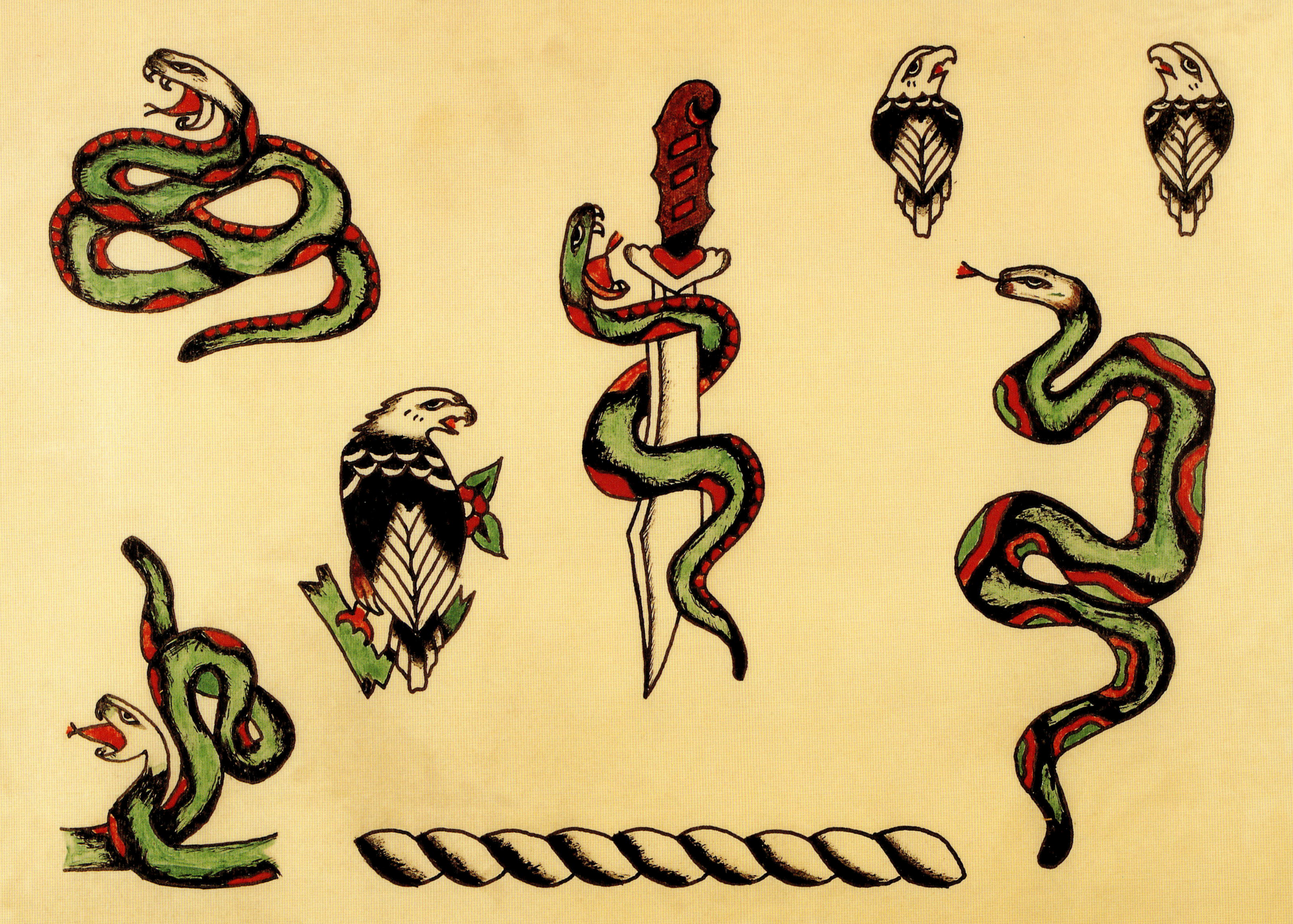

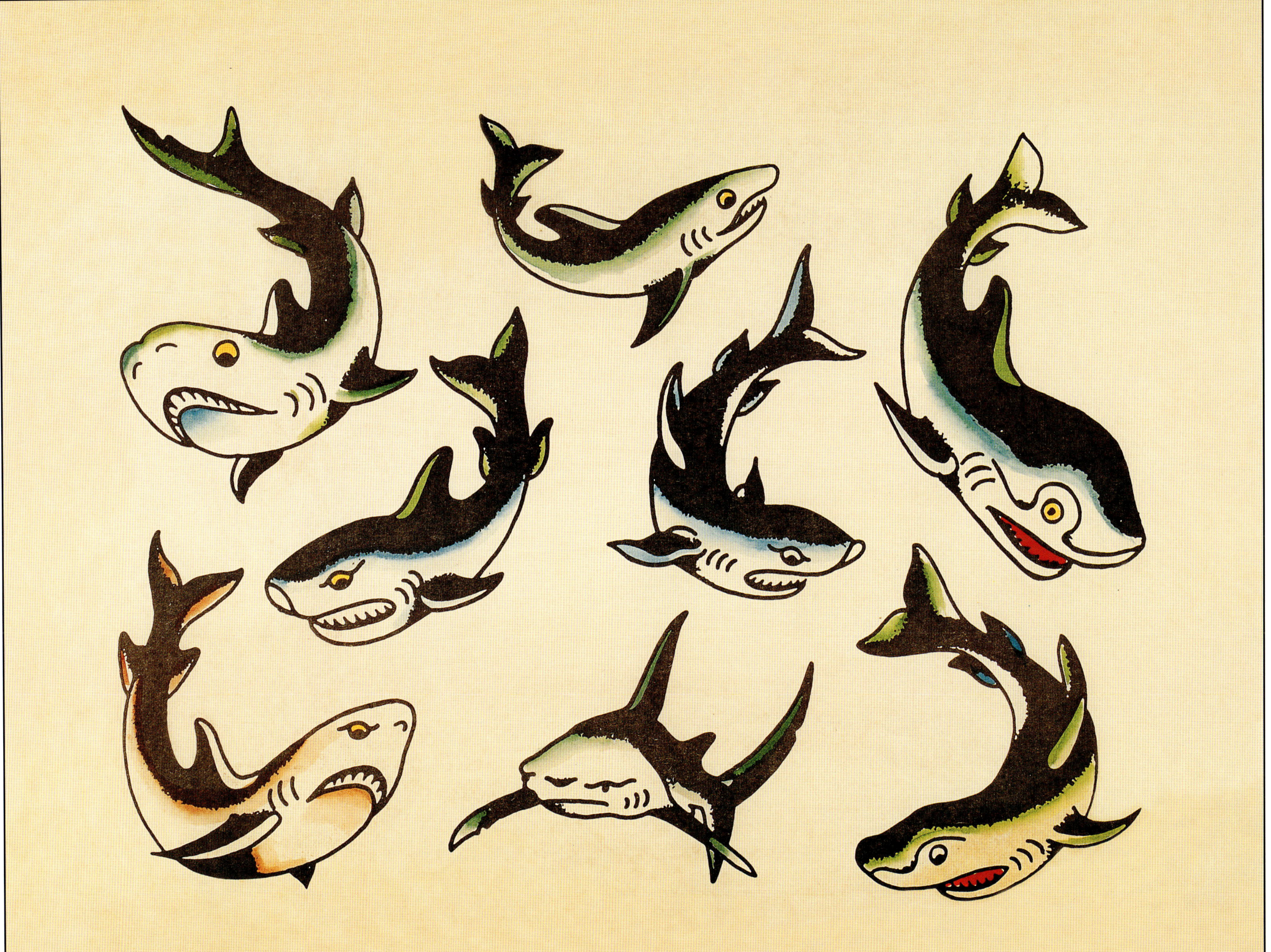

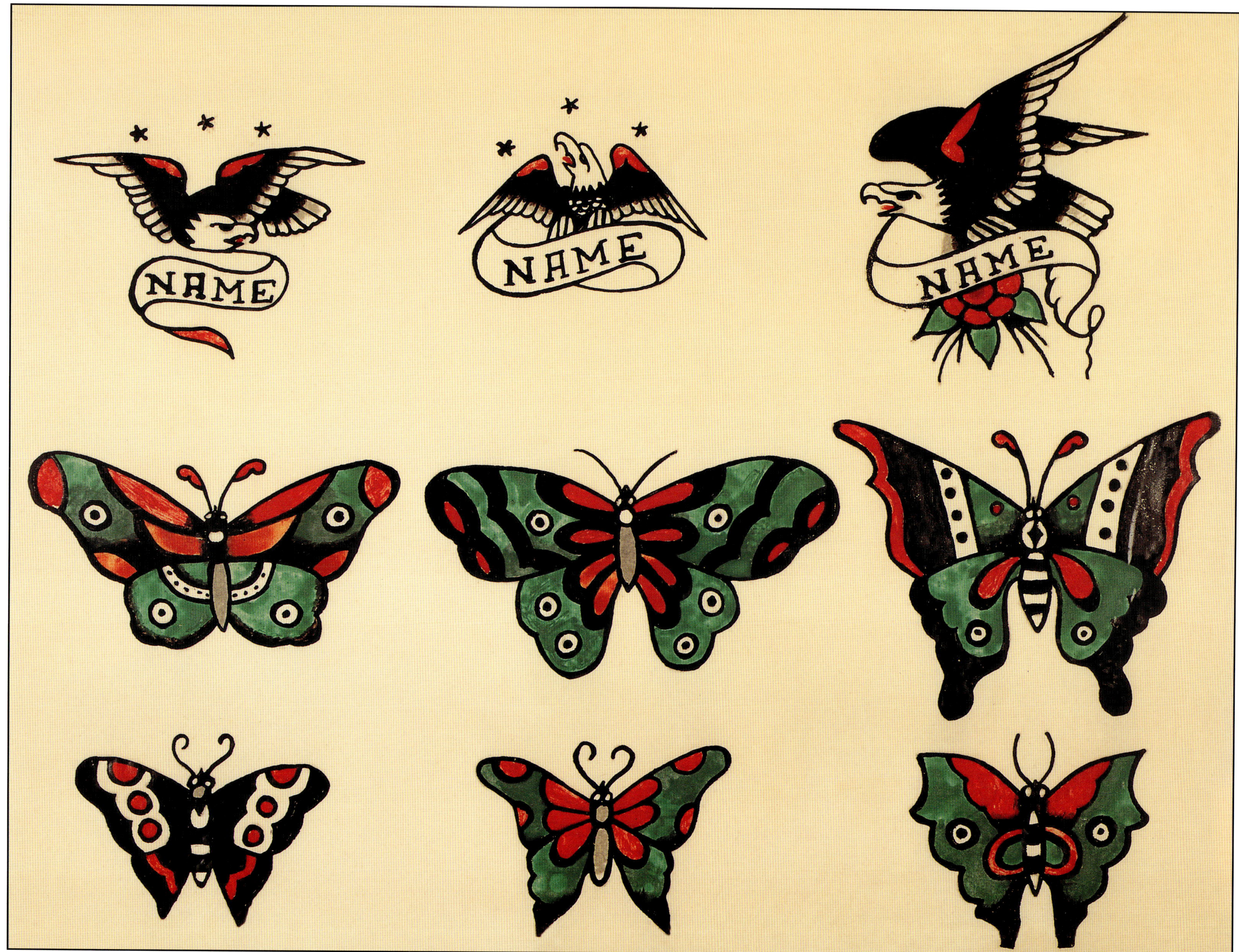
NAME
NAME
NAME

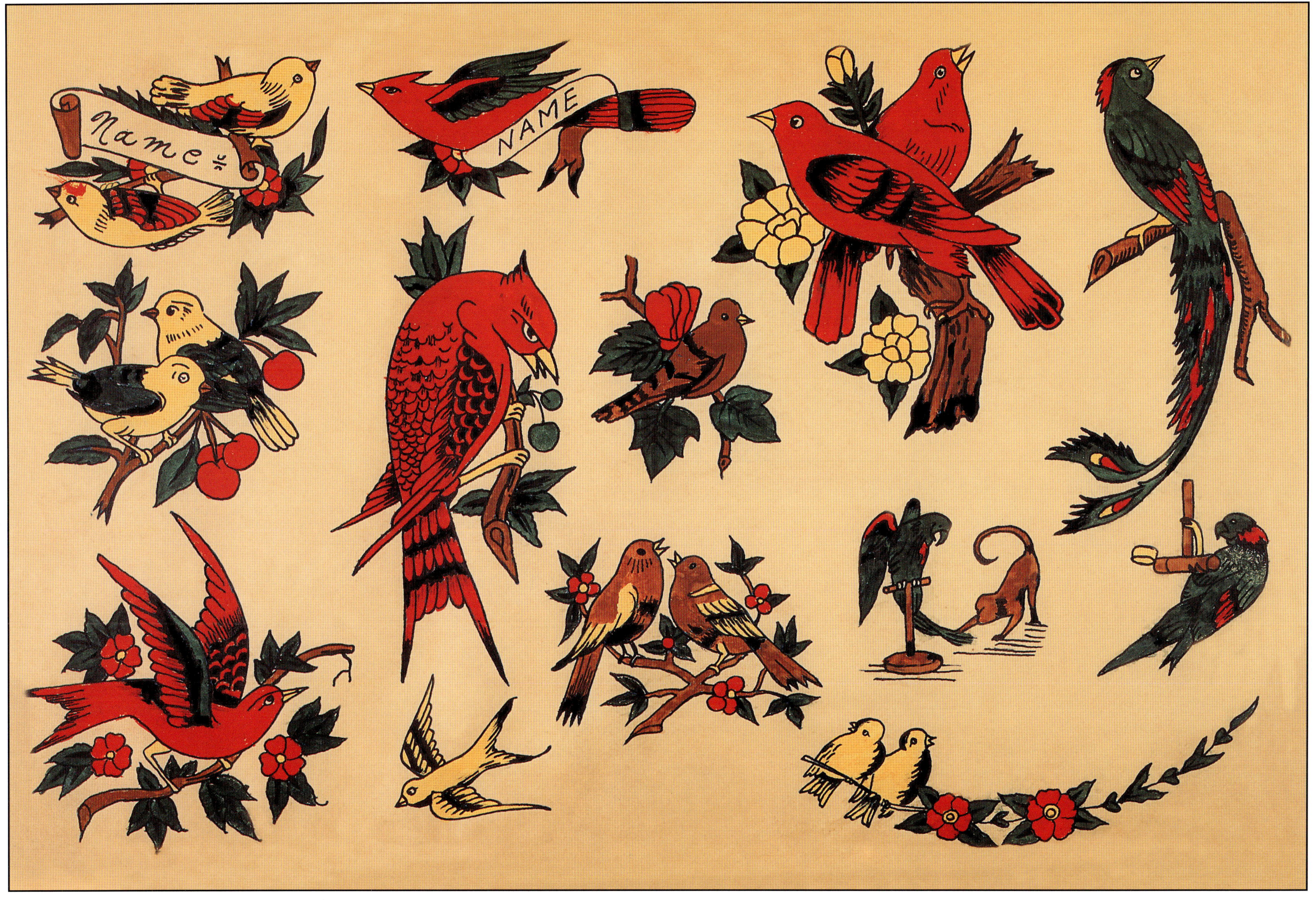

Name
NAME

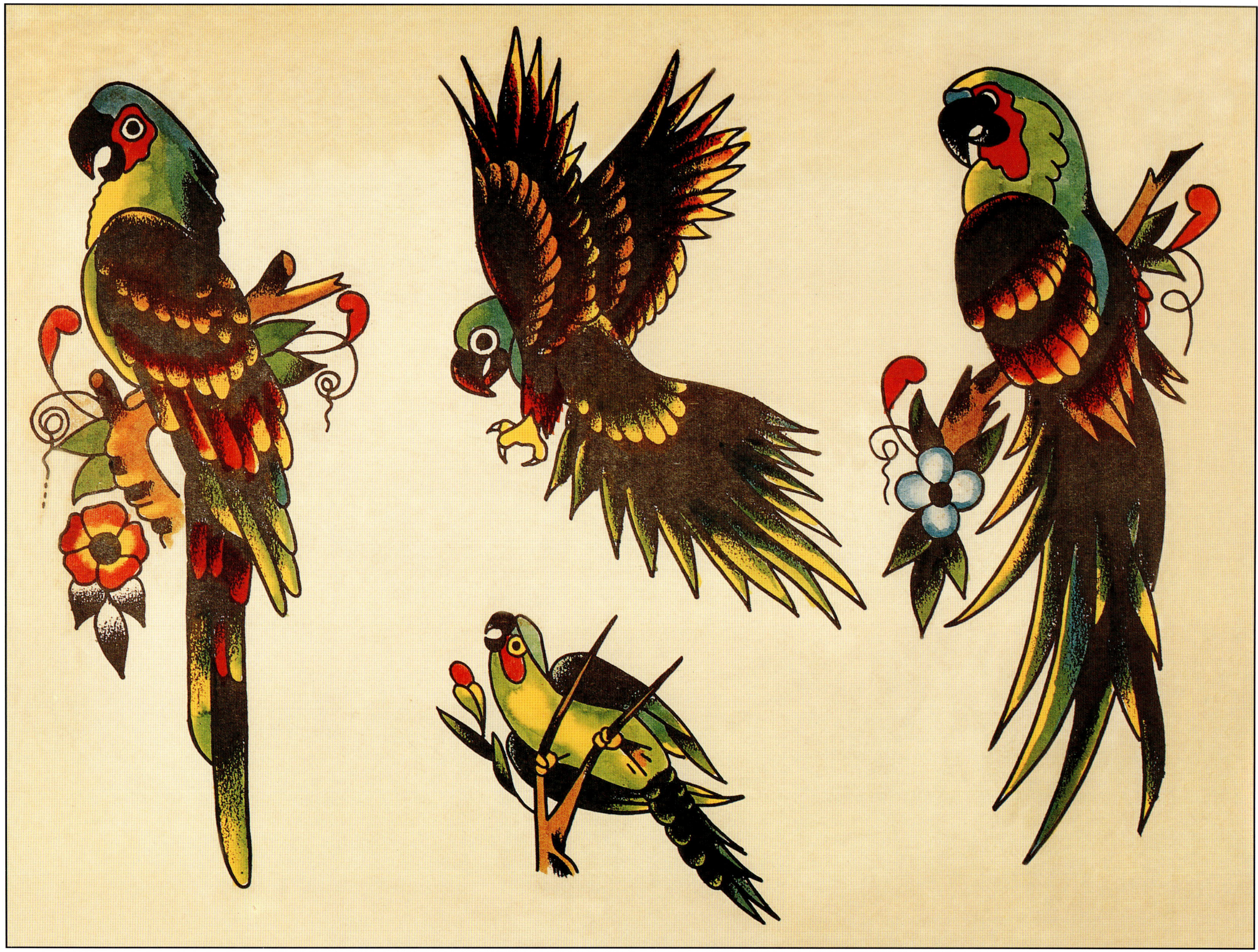

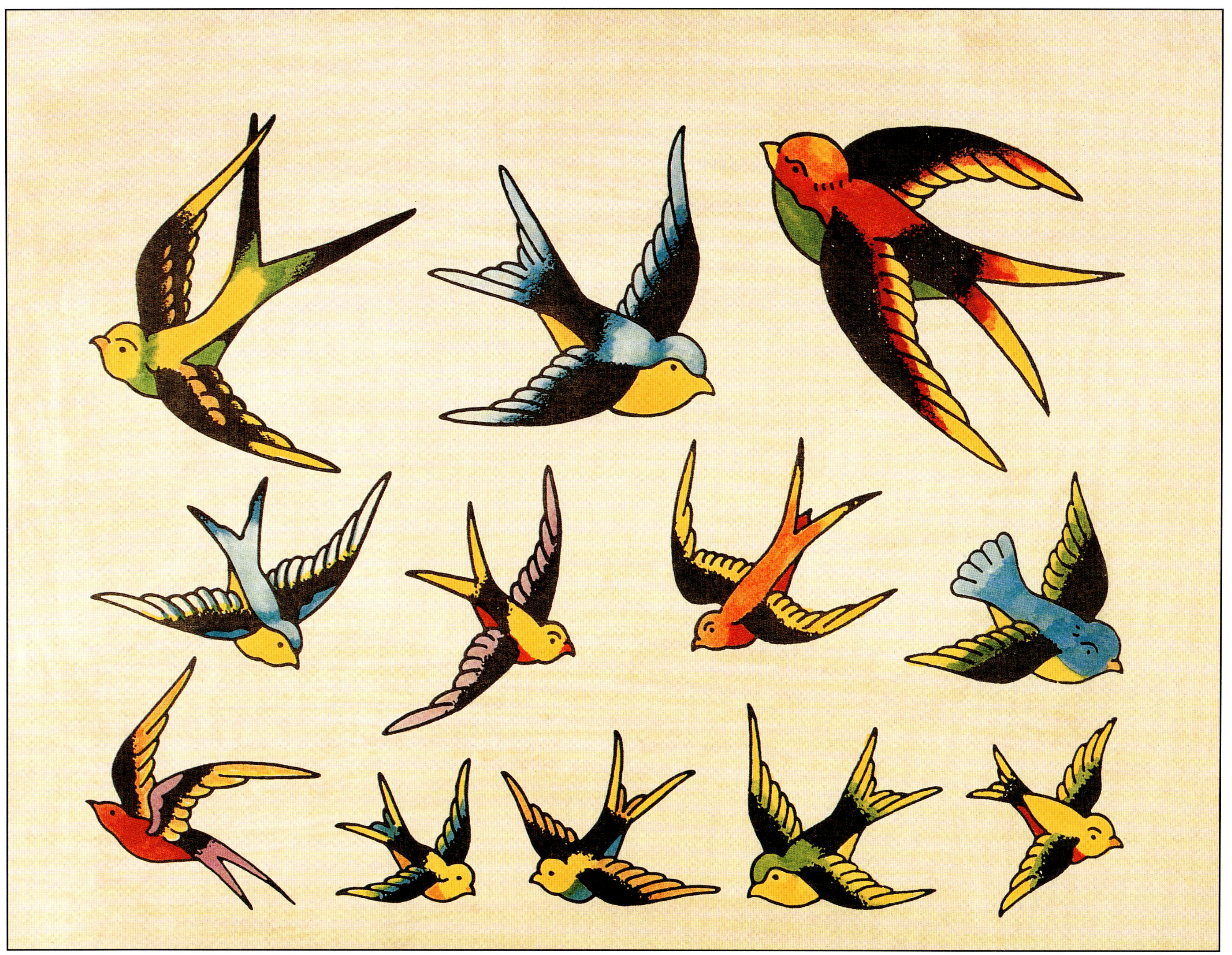

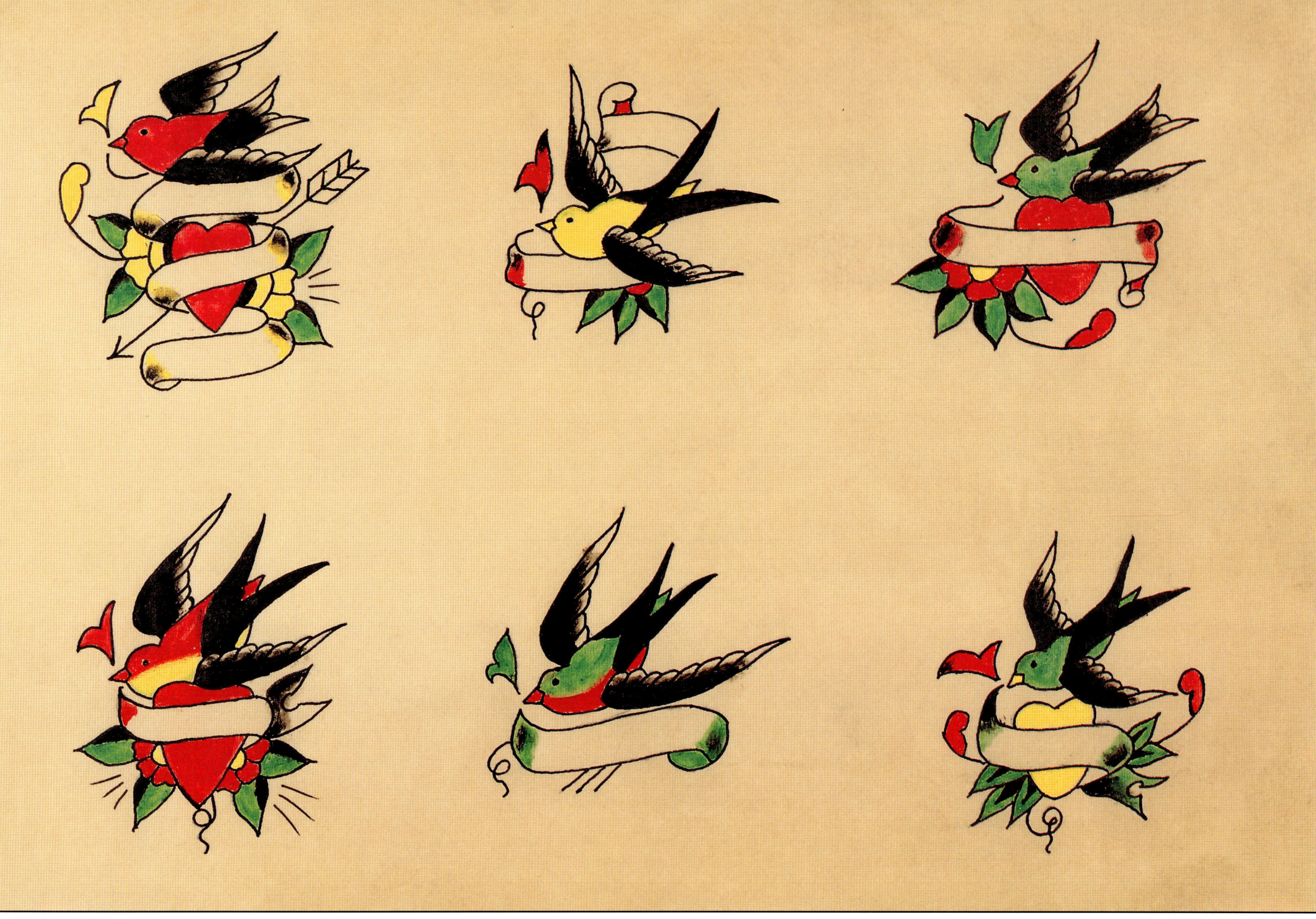